FACULTY DEVELOPMENT WORKBOOK

MODULE 3:
TECHNIQUES FOR
CLASSROOM PRESENTATION

FACULTY DEVELOPMENT WORKBOOK

MODULE 3:
TECHNIQUES FOR
CLASSROOM PRESENTATION

Amy Solomon, MS, OTR

Quantum Integrations

THOMSON

DELMAR LEARNING   Australia Brazil Canada Mexico Singapore Spain United Kingdom United States

THOMSON

DELMAR LEARNING

Faculty Development Workbook
Module 3: Techniques for Classroom Presentation

Amy Solomon, MS, OTR
Quantum Integrations

Vice President, Career Education SBU:
Dawn Gerrain

Acquisitions Editor:
Martine Edwards

Managing Editor:
Robert L. Serenka, Jr.

Developmental Editor:
Jennifer Anderson

Editorial Assistant:
Falon Ferraro

Director of Production:
Wendy A. Troeger

Production Manager:
J.P. Henkel

Content Project Manager:
Amber Leith

Director of Marketing:
Wendy E. Mapstone

Channel Manager:
Kristin McNary

Compositor:
Interactive Composition Corporation

ISBN: 1-4180-3725-7
ISBN: 978-1-4180-3725-3

NOTICE TO THE READER

CONTENTS

SECTION 3   Effective Questioning Techniques   77

SECTION 4   Effective Lecture Techniques   111

SECTION 5   Effective Discussion Techniques   145

INTRODUCTION

DELMAR'S FACULTY DEVELOPMENT SERIES

Delmar's Faculty Development Series consists of a collection of online courses covering a wide range of topics relevant to contemporary education and the development of quality teaching practices. In addition to course content, the online courses offer added value through features that support practical application of the material, including reflection questions, activities, ideas for classroom activities and assignments, professional portfolio development, and a tool for setting and tracking professional development goals.

HOW TO USE THIS WORKBOOK

The Faculty Development Workbook is offered as a guide and supplement to the main online course. Each workbook is customized to the content of its corresponding online course and is intended to customize the online content to individual needs. Because access to the online component has time constraints, completing each module's corresponding workbook provides a permanent reference for material once access to the online course has expired. Completing the workbook will provide you with a guide that includes a "refresher" course of material covered, ideas for development of your curriculum and courses over time, and methods for continued development of your teaching skills.

Workbook Components and Their Applications

Each workbook contains elements that correspond to the items found in its corresponding online course. Before using the workbook, take the time to understand how each element can be used to support you in completing the online course and to develop a resource for future reference.

Main Headings

Each of the main headings found in the online course is represented in the workbook. Space is provided for you to make notes of important concepts, ideas, and most importantly, to customize the information to your own needs. These notes will be your main resource after your access time to the online course has expired, so using this feature to its maximum potential will be of great benefit in the future.

Take It to the Classroom Activities

Take It to the Classroom activities are learning activities for you to use in your classroom with students. They are designed to provide you with specific activities that you can use immediately in the classroom and to help you apply the concepts of the online course. Some activities may be more appropriate for your group of students than others, and you are encouraged to select activities that fit your needs. One benefit of having the completed workbook is that you will be able to refer back to and select different activities as you teach classes with various needs each term. Space for planning each activity is provided. The online component provides the background needed to meet the goal of each activity.

Learning Activities

The Learning Activities provided at the conclusion of each section are capstone activities intended to synthesize the concepts from the section and provide an opportunity to apply them in practical situations. Activities include individual, group, and online formats, and the background needed to meet the goal of each activity is provided in the online component.

Activity Files

Throughout the online courses, activities are provided to illustrate main concepts, support the development of teaching skills, and conduct assessments of goal achievement. Completion of the Activity Files supports achievement of section learning objectives. The goals of these activities are also supported by online course content, and their successful completion provides the foundation for the capstone learning activities at the end of each section. Activity sheets and instructions are provided in both the online course and in the workbook.

Learning Objectives Revisited

Learning objectives are listed at the beginning of each section. Mastery of the online content and completion of the reflection questions and activities contribute to the achievement of the objectives. Learning Objectives Revisited provides you with a tool for assessing your own learning and setting goals for future development in areas covered in the section. The completed workbook will be a valuable resource to you in achieving this goal after your access to the online course has expired.

Instructor Improvement Plan

The Instructor Improvement Plan is designed as a long-term professional development tool. It provides a mechanism for setting individual goals in areas important to your professional development. The tool provides a means for recording goals, time frames, and methods for completion, as well as the opportunity to modify goals over time. One Instructor Improvement Plan form is provided for each module. You are encouraged to make a copy for each section and set individual goals for each section. You may wish to use this tool as part of your school's professional development and faculty assessment program.

Professional Development Portfolio

The Professional Development Portfolio is a collection of learning activities that you have completed and that serve as documentation of your professional development. Portfolios can be used as records of your professional development or to document your achievements to supervisors or other professional colleagues. Each module provides a guide for creating a Professional Development Portfolio based on module content. You are encouraged to modify this guide as necessary to support your interests and needs.

SECTION

1

EFFECTIVE PRESENTATION TECHNIQUES

LEARNING OBJECTIVES

Upon successful completion of Section 1, the instructor will have achieved the following objectives. Check off each of the objectives as you have mastered it. You will have the opportunity to assess your performance on each objective at the end of Section 1.

1. The instructor will identify important elements of a successful and unsuccessful presentation, analyze his or her presentation technique, and make suggestions for personal improvement.

INTRODUCTORY QUESTIONS

- What concerns, fears, responsibilities, likes, dislikes, and frustrations do people have about speaking or presenting in public? How do you personally manage these factors when teaching students?
- What things affect your own confidence level before a presentation?
- Think back to the best and the worst presentation you have given or have observed. What made the difference in the two outcomes?
- What feedback have you received from peers or students about your presentation technique? (Check your recent faculty evaluations.)
- How receptive to presentations are your students? In general, when do students seem most receptive to an instructor's presentation?

OVERVIEW

Section 1 covers several topics about effective presentations, including using delivery techniques, establishing rapport with students, capturing and keeping students' attention, using various types of visual aids, and applying techniques for developing presentation skills.

SUGGESTED GENERAL GUIDELINES: DELIVERY TECHNIQUES

Compare two presentations that you have made. How did the two presentations differ? What made them effective or ineffective?

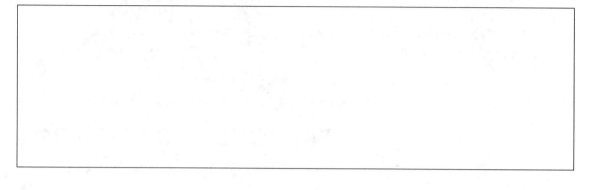

■ ■ ■ DIVERSITY CONSIDERATIONS ■ ■ ■

 As much as possible, learn about students' disabilities or special needs ahead of time so you can make the necessary accommodations.

DIVERSITY REFLECTIONS

- What types of accommodations might you make for a student with a hearing impairment? With a visual impairment?

The Audience

Note ways in which your audience has influenced your delivery techniques.

REFLECTION QUESTIONS

Be sure to record your answers to these questions in the space provided and file them in the appropriate section of your Professional Development Portfolio.

- What do you know about your students that you can use in the development of classroom activities?

_____

_____

_____

_____

_____

- What things would you like to find out that would be helpful in your teaching?

_____

_____

_____

_____

_____

- What is your preferred method for obtaining this information?

_____

_____

_____

_____

_____

The Physical Environment

Make an assessment of the physical environment in your classroom(s) according to the criteria in the online course. How might the physical environment be improved?

See the *Physical Environment Checklist* found at the end of this section.

The Material

How has your course material affected your delivery technique or style?

```
┌─────────────────────────────────────────────────────────────┐
│                                                             │
│                                                             │
│                                                             │
│                                                             │
│                                                             │
│                                                             │
└─────────────────────────────────────────────────────────────┘
```

REFLECTION QUESTIONS

Be sure to record your answers to these questions in the space provided and file them in the appropriate section of your Professional Development Portfolio.

- Where is the material in your course(s) complex, emotional, ambiguous, and/or controversial?

_____

_____

_____

_____

_____

- What can you do to facilitate the learning with each different type of content?

_____

_____

_____

_____

_____

The Instructor or Presenter

What are your typical presentation methods? How effective are they?

```
┌─────────────────────────────────────────────────────────────┐
│                                                             │
│                                                             │
│                                                             │
│                                                             │
│                                                             │
│                                                             │
└─────────────────────────────────────────────────────────────┘
```

See the *Peer Review/Instructor Observation Form—Presentation Style* found at the end of this section.

REFLECTION QUESTIONS

Be sure to record your answers to these questions in the space provided and file them in the appropriate section of your Professional Development Portfolio.

- What do you see as your classroom presentation strengths?

_____

_____

_____

_____

_____

- What do you see as your weaknesses?

_____

_____

_____

_____

_____

- What areas would you like to improve?

_____

_____

_____

_____

_____

_____

ESTABLISHING RAPPORT WITH STUDENTS

How do you currently establish rapport with students? What techniques are most effective? How would you like to improve? Under each of the following headings, record what you currently do to use that strategy in your classes. Also, list methods for developing your skills in that area. Add other categories as needed.

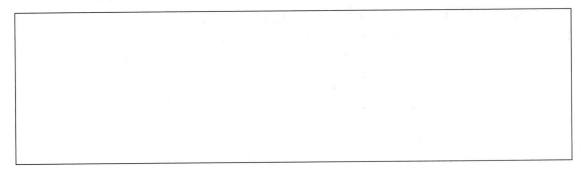

■ ■ ■ DIVERSITY CONSIDERATIONS ■ ■ ■

Acceptable methods for establishing rapport may vary cross-culturally. Be sensitive to students of diverse backgrounds who may not be comfortable with Western practices. Establish rapport in a manner that supports their level of comfort.

DIVERSITY REFLECTIONS

- How do you typically establish rapport with students?

_____

_____

_____

_____

_____

- How can you tell if a student is uncomfortable with your approach? How do you address the situation?

_____

_____

_____

_____

_____

_____

Greet Students

Stay after Class to Chat with Students

Be Available Outside of Class

Interact More and Lecture Less

Make Eye Contact

■ ■ DIVERSITY CONSIDERATIONS ■ ■ ■

Eye contact is an example of interpersonal behavior that varies cross-culturally. In some cultures, it is considered rude to make eye contact with a figure of authority such as a teacher.

DIVERSITY REFLECTIONS

- Eye contact is considered an important part of nonverbal communication in Western culture. How would you respect a cultural difference while preparing a student for the Western workplace?

_____

_____

_____

_____

_____

Avoid Using Filler Words

Don't Read or Recite Your Notes in Class

Look at Students When They Speak

Read Students' Nonverbal Messages

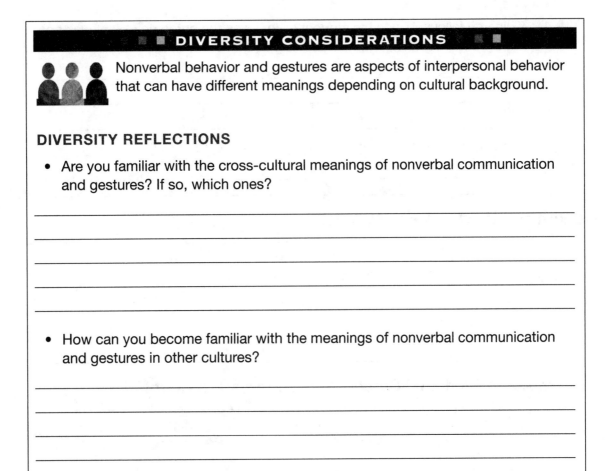

■ ■ DIVERSITY CONSIDERATIONS ■ ■

Nonverbal behavior and gestures are aspects of interpersonal behavior that can have different meanings depending on cultural background.

DIVERSITY REFLECTIONS

- Are you familiar with the cross-cultural meanings of nonverbal communication and gestures? If so, which ones?

_____

_____

_____

_____

_____

- How can you become familiar with the meanings of nonverbal communication and gestures in other cultures?

_____

_____

_____

_____

_____

REFLECTION QUESTIONS

Be sure to record your answers to these questions in the space provided and file them in the appropriate section of your Professional Development Portfolio.

- What other expressions and nonverbal behavior have you observed in your classes?

_____

_____

_____

_____

- What did these communicate to you as an instructor? Did you clarify the meaning with the student? Were your perceptions accurate?

_____

_____

_____

_____

- How did you follow up with the student? What was the outcome? What was positive about the resolution, and what would you do differently?

_____

_____

_____

_____

_____

Learn and Use Students' Names

Learn About Students' Career Goals, Interests, and Hobbies

Familiarize Yourself with Students' Fields of Study

REFLECTION QUESTIONS

Be sure to record your answers to these questions in the space provided and file them in the appropriate section of your Professional Development Portfolio.

- What fields of study are represented in the classes you are currently teaching?

_____

_____

_____

_____

- What questions can you research or ask to learn more about each field's interface with your discipline?

_____

_____

_____

_____

_____

Smile

Share Stories

REFLECTION QUESTIONS

Be sure to record your answers to these questions in the space provided and file them in the appropriate section of your Professional Development Portfolio.

- Can you think of a time you successfully shared a story with your class and a time when sharing was unsuccessful?

_____

_____

_____

_____

- How were the two situations different?

_____

_____

_____

_____

_____

Crack a Joke

REFLECTION QUESTIONS

Be sure to record your answers to these questions in the space provided and file them in the appropriate section of your Professional Development Portfolio.

- What other techniques have you used successfully to develop rapport with students? (Also, list techniques you have observed or heard about from your colleagues. Consider adding the development of new rapport-building techniques to your Instructor Improvement Plan).

_____

_____

_____

_____

_____

CAPTURING STUDENTS' ATTENTION

What catches your students' attention? What attention grabbers are most effective? How might you improve your expertise in capturing students' attention? Under each of the following headings, record what you currently do to use that strategy in your classes. Also, list methods for developing your skills in that area. Add other categories as needed.

Introduce Your Topic by Sharing an Unusual Object

Begin with Startling or Interesting Statistics

Begin with an Activity or Demonstration

Show a Film Clip

Start with a Joke

Discuss a Current Issue

[blank box]

See the *Attention Grabbers Brainstorming Worksheet* at the end of this section.

REFLECTION QUESTIONS

Be sure to record your answers to these questions in the space provided and file them in the appropriate section of your Professional Development Portfolio.

- What successful techniques have you used or observed for grabbing learner attention?

_____

_____

_____

_____

_____

- For which topics do you need to beef up your attention-grabbing techniques?

_____

_____

_____

_____

_____

KEEPING STUDENTS' ATTENTION

What keeps students' attention? How successfully do you currently keep their attention? How might you improve? Under each of the following headings, record what you currently do to use that strategy in your classes. Also, list ideas for developing skills in that area. Add additional categories as needed.

[blank box]

Pace Yourself

Project Outwardly to Your Audience

Avoid Negative Nonverbal Behaviors

REFLECTION QUESTIONS

Be sure to record your answers to these questions in the space provided and file them in the appropriate section of your Professional Development Portfolio.

- What is the most annoying nonverbal mannerism you have observed in your academic career?

_____

_____

_____

_____

_____

- Which areas of nonverbal behavior can you improve? What feedback have you received on instructor evaluations about any distracting behaviors?

_____

_____

_____

_____

_____

- What can you do to break any "bad habits" that may be distracting your students?

_____

_____

_____

_____

_____

GENERAL TECHNIQUES FOR USING VISUAL AIDS

What visual aids do you currently use? How effective are they? For each of the headings that follow, comment on how well your use of visual aids meets the criterion.

Use Visual Aids Only When They Add to Your Presentation

Use Appropriate Visual Aids

DIVERSITY CONSIDERATIONS

When planning visual aids, consider the needs of students with visual impairments and the needs of older students. Older students may need brighter light while avoiding glare. Consider these needs when setting up visual aids.

DIVERSITY REFLECTIONS

- How could you adjust your classroom lighting to maximize brightness and minimize glare?

_____

_____

_____

_____

_____

Make Each Visual Aid Stand on Its Own

REFLECTION QUESTIONS

Be sure to record your answers to these questions in the space provided and file them in the appropriate section of your Professional Development Portfolio.

- Which visual aids that fit the preceding criteria could you use in a class you are teaching?

_____

_____

_____

_____

_____

- Ask a student to review one of your visual aids for clarity and ease of under-standing. Does it meet the criteria listed above?

_____

_____

_____

_____

_____

Design the Layout of Visual Aids Carefully

See the *Visual Aid Review Form* at the end of this section.

Check the Room and Available Equipment

Know How to Use the Equipment

Be sure to record your answers to these questions in the space provided and file them in the appropriate section of your Professional Development Portfolio.

- What specific equipment is available for use in the classroom?

_____

_____

_____

_____

_____

- What are the usage policies and procedures?

_____

_____

_____

_____

_____

- Is there specific equipment available that you are not using? Why are you not using it and how can you learn how to use it?

_____

_____

_____

_____

_____

Keep It Simple

REFLECTION QUESTIONS

Be sure to record your answers to these questions in the space provided and file them in the appropriate section of your Professional Development Portfolio.

- Do your visual aids fit the description of simplicity in the online course?

_____

_____

_____

_____

_____

- What can you change to simplify your visual aids? (Write a brief critique and suggest improvements. Consider seeking the input of other instructors in your program or department.)

_____

_____

_____

_____

_____

Avoid Distracting from the Presentation

Proofread the Visual Aids

Interact with Your Students, Not with the Visual Aid

Avoid Relying on Visuals for an Opening

Avoid Using Visuals in Closing

Graph Technical Data

REFLECTION QUESTIONS

Be sure to record your answers to these questions in the space provided and file them in the appropriate section of your Professional Development Portfolio.

- Which format is most effective and why?

_____

_____

_____

_____

_____

- What other types of data do you share with students? What do you think would be the most effective visual for this data? Why? (Consider what you learned from creating several types of graphs and charts in answering this part of the question.)

_____

_____

_____

_____

_____

Control Your Visuals

REFLECTION QUESTIONS

Be sure to record your answers to these questions in the space provided and file them in the appropriate section of your Professional Development Portfolio.

- What is the worst visual aid "disaster" you can recall?

_____

_____

_____

_____

_____

- What are your personal pet peeves about visual aids—either using or observing?

_____

_____

_____

_____

_____

_____

TYPES OF VISUAL AIDS

Consider the types of visual aids presented in the online course. For each type listed below, note the advantages and disadvantages that the aid might present for your classes. Record ideas for its use for each class. Take into account the considerations made in the online course for each type of visual aid.

Computer-Based Presentation Software

Overhead Projectors

Slide Projectors and 35mm Slides

Electronic Whiteboards

Posters and Flip Charts

Videos

Handouts

Samples, Examples, and Demonstrations

Chalkboard or Whiteboard

DVDs

See the *Visual Aid Worksheet* at the end of this section.

REFLECTION QUESTIONS

Be sure to record your answers to these questions in the space provided and file them in the appropriate section of your Professional Development Portfolio.

- What visuals do you use most in your teaching? Why?

_____

_____

_____

_____

_____

- What other visual aids could you use to enhance your presentations?

_____

_____

_____

_____

_____

IMPROVING YOUR DELIVERY TECHNIQUE

What resources do you have available that might be useful to you in developing your delivery techniques?

Consider these resources and techniques as you review the following headings. For each heading, devise a strategy that would be helpful to you in developing your delivery expertise in the classroom. Use the information in the online component to guide you in formulating your ideas and responses.

Practice, Practice, Practice

Get Additional Training

REFLECTION QUESTIONS

Be sure to record your answers to these questions in the space provided and file them in the appropriate section of your Professional Development Portfolio.

Compare a time in the classroom when you felt prepared and confident, versus a time when you did not.

- What was different about your level of preparation?

_____

_____

_____

_____

_____

- What other factors may have contributed to your feelings of confidence, or lack thereof?

_____

_____

_____

_____

_____

Critique Yourself

Develop a Plan of Action

See the *Teaching Development Review Form* at the end of this section.

Implement Your Action Plan

Reevaluate Yourself

LEARNING ACTIVITIES

The following activities are designed to support you in applying the module concepts to your teaching activities. Use the "Notes for Planning This Activity" spaces to record your ideas and to note resources. Complete each activity and submit as directed by your campus faculty development director. File copies of your activities and any evaluation comments you receive in your Professional Development Portfolio.

Lecture Planning Worksheet

 Develop a worksheet you can use to plan the lectures for your course. Complete this activity in groups of three to five instructors.

Notes for Planning This Activity:

Lecture Assessment

 Use your Lecture Planning Worksheet to evaluate the different elements of a lecture you have presented in the past or a lecture presented by a colleague in a college course. Make recommendations for improvement.

Complete this evaluation in groups of three to four instructors, preferably who teach in similar areas.

Notes for Planning This Activity:

Lecture Development Activity

For a course you are or will be teaching, develop a topical lecture using the techniques discussed. Use your Lecture Planning Worksheet.

Notes for Planning This Activity:

LEARNING OBJECTIVES REVISITED

Review the Learning Objectives for Section 1 and rate your level of achievement for each objective using the rating scale provided. Following your assessment, determine the steps you need to take to meet the objective effectively. For each objective on which you do not rate yourself as a 3, outline a plan of action that you will take to achieve the objective fully. Include a time frame for this plan. Review completed Learning Activities for specific areas in which you need further development. Include the assessment and goals that you write in your Professional Development Portfolio. You may wish to use the Instructor Improvement Plan to set goals to further work toward learning objectives.

1 = did not successfully achieve objective
2 = understand what is needed, but need more study or practice
3 = achieved learning objective thoroughly

	1	2	3
1. The instructor will identify important elements of a successful and unsuccessful presentation, analyze his or her presentation technique, and make suggestions for personal improvement.	☐	☐	☐

STEPS TO ACHIEVE UNMET OBJECTIVES

Steps	Date
1. _____	_____
2. _____	_____
3. _____	_____
4. _____	_____

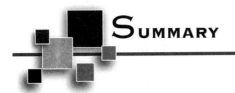 **S**UMMARY

Section 1 discussed numerous techniques for audience presentations, specifically for the college classroom. You read about basic delivery techniques plus ideas for assessing and improving your delivery technique. You learned tips for using instructional media and visual aids. You should now be able to identify good presentation techniques, identify areas in which you are strong, and improve areas in which you need further work.

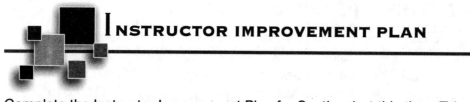

INSTRUCTOR IMPROVEMENT PLAN

Complete the Instructor Improvement Plan for Section 1 at this time. Take the necessary time to prepare a thoughtful, detailed improvement plan. Complete the form and keep it available as you plan and teach your classes for the next few terms. Note your progress, problems, successes, and questions over the next three to six months. At that time, reevaluate the plan and set new goals. Depending on the format you have selected for your Professional Development Portfolio, file the elements of your instructional plan in the appropriate sections. Record the dates for reassessing your goals on the professional development schedule at the beginning of your portfolio.

PROFESSIONAL DEVELOPMENT PORTFOLIO ELEMENTS

To finish Section 1, insert your completed responses, reflections, and activities from the section into the designated parts of your Professional Development Portfolio.

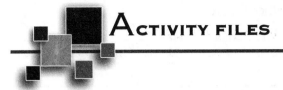

ACTIVITY FILES

The activities on the following pages will help you achieve the Section 1 learning objectives that are referenced throughout the section. In the online module, there are links to PDF files with supporting documents or worksheets for these activities.

PHYSICAL ENVIRONMENT CHECKLIST

Instructions: Use this form to evaluate your classroom's physical environment or another environment in which you may deliver a presentation. Note any improvements that might enhance the physical learning environment. Some areas may be fairly simple to change, while others may be a bit more challenging. Remember, there is usually more than one way to accomplish something. For example, it might not be feasible to change a lighting system, but desks and tables can be rearranged to reduce or eliminate glare. Be creative!

■ Are there visual or auditory distractions (including the drone of air conditioning and heating vents)?

_____

_____

_____

_____

_____

■ Do the air conditioning/heating vents blow directly on any of the seating areas?

_____

_____

_____

_____

_____

■ Is the temperature well regulated?

_____

_____

_____

_____

_____

■ Is the lighting of an appropriate intensity, without glare?

_____

_____

_____

_____

_____

■ Does the seating arrangement allow for unobstructed vision and hearing?

_____

_____

_____

_____

_____

■ Is the seating arrangement appropriate for the activity?

_____

_____

_____

_____

_____

■ Can the seating be modified to better suit the activity? How?

_____

_____

_____

_____

_____

PEER REVIEW/INSTRUCTOR OBSERVATION FORM— PRESENTATION STYLE

Use this form for observation by a faculty member, your faculty training coordinator, or other professional colleague at your school. Remember to use any feedback that you receive in your Instructor Improvement Plan.

Date: _____ Class: _____

Comment on the general presentation style. Please be specific and give examples.

_____

_____

_____

_____

_____

_____

_____

How did this skill affect class dynamics and the activity? Please be as specific as possible.

_____

_____

_____

_____

_____

_____

_____

Please comment on specific elements, such as timing, physical and emotional environment of the classroom, and appropriateness of materials to the content. Add other elements as you see fit.

_____

_____

_____

_____

_____

_____

_____

Based on the goals of the activity and the responses of the class, how effective were the presentation skills?

_____

_____

_____

_____

_____

_____

_____

How could the presentation skills be developed to further facilitate the class dynamic and activity?

_____

_____

_____

_____

_____

_____

_____

_____

Other Comments: _____

_____

_____

_____

_____

_____

ATTENTION GRABBERS BRAINSTORMING WORKSHEET

Instructions: For the categories below, identify specific items in your field that could be used to capture students' attention. Remember that some element of surprise or unexpectedness adds to the effectiveness of this technique. Also—be outrageous! Have fun! At this point, don't limit yourself by expense, availability, or other practical concerns. Even if you can't get exactly what you record here, your responses may generate more feasible ideas.

■ Unusual Objects

_____

_____

_____

_____

_____

■ Startling or Unusual Statistics

_____

_____

_____

_____

_____

■ Activities or Demonstrations

_____

_____

_____

_____

_____

■ Film Clips

_____

_____

_____

_____

_____

■ Jokes

_____

_____

_____

_____

_____

■ Current Events and Issues

_____

_____

_____

_____

_____

VISUAL AID REVIEW

Instructions: Design a visual aid for a class that you are teaching, or will be teaching. Be sure to consider the design recommendations discussed in the module. Upon completion, present the aid to a student or colleague. Ask them to fill in this review form by commenting on the items below. Request that they respond to the visual aid from the perspective of a student in class. Then, compare their reactions with the recommended design guidelines.

DESIGN ELEMENT	COMMENTS	SUGGESTIONS
Use of Fonts		
Use of Color		
Transitions		
Use of Space		
Focus on Main Points		

VISUAL AID WORKSHEET

 Instructions: For one of the classes you are teaching, or will be teaching, consider the information you will provide students. Decide:

- Which information will best be presented using a visual aid (Activity)?
- Which type of visual aid would best convey the information (Type of Visual Aid)?
- Why you chose this particular type (Rationale)?

Remember that there may be information that is not best conveyed with visual aids. The goal of completing this worksheet is to determine what information benefits most from visual aids and the type of visual aid that is best suited for the task. If a visual aid does not seem to be the best choice, consider another method. You may find it helpful to complete this activity with other instructors from your program or department.

Class: _____

Activity	Type of Visual Aid	Rationale
_____	_____	_____
_____	_____	_____
_____	_____	_____
_____	_____	_____
_____	_____	_____
_____	_____	_____
_____	_____	_____
_____	_____	_____
_____	_____	_____
_____	_____	_____
_____	_____	_____
_____	_____	_____
_____	_____	_____
_____	_____	_____

TEACHING DEVELOPMENT REVIEW PLAN

Instructor: Use this form for regular observation by members of your professional development group. Maintain completed reviews so you can see your progress over time. Remember to use any feedback that you receive in setting additional goals. This is intended to be an ongoing process. Remember to incorporate this feedback into your plan for ongoing professional development.

Reviewer: Please be as specific as possible by giving examples of observed behavior whenever possible. Feel free to make suggestions for skill development.

Date: _____ Class: _____

How well did the instructor prepare the physical environment and materials?

_____

_____

_____

_____

How did the instructor demonstrate awareness of the students in the audience?

_____

_____

_____

_____

How did the instructor establish and maintain rapport with the students?

_____

_____

_____

_____

How did the instructor capture and hold students' attention and interest throughout the presentation?

_____

_____

_____

_____

Comment on the use of visual aids. Were the visuals effective for conveying the information? Did the instructor use them as successfully as possible? If so, what was most effective? What could have been improved?

_____

_____

_____

_____

_____

Other Comments:

_____

_____

_____

_____

_____

PRESENTATION EVALUATION FORM

  Develop a detailed evaluation form that you can use to evaluate your own presentation techniques as well as those of your colleagues. Be sure it is detailed enough to describe the presentation sufficiently to recommend improvements. This activity should be completed in groups of three to five instructors.

Notes for Planning This Activity:

PRESENTATION CRITIQUE ACTIVITY

Critique three educational presentations from videotapes or in person, perhaps using colleagues who agree to be taped. Identify the positive and negative behaviors covered in this section and recommend improvements. Use the Presentation Evaluation Form from the previous activity.

Notes for Planning This Activity:

PRESENTATION SELF-ASSESSMENT ACTIVITY

Videotape at least two of your own lectures. Identify your positive and negative presentation behaviors and develop a plan of action for improvement.

Notes for Planning This Activity:

SECTION

2

EFFECTIVE LISTENING TECHNIQUES

LEARNING OBJECTIVES

Upon successful completion of Section 2, the instructor will have achieved the following objectives. Check off each of the objectives as you have mastered it. You will have the opportunity to assess your performance on each objective at the end of Section 2.

2. The instructor will demonstrate the ability to use effective listening techniques in a classroom setting, including demonstrating the ability to understand a question before answering it, making students feel respected and valued, and showing a willingness to listen sincerely.

3. The instructor will demonstrate the ability to identify motives behind student questions and make appropriate responses to their concerns.

INTRODUCTORY QUESTIONS

- On what occasions do you feel that others truly listen to you?
- How do you feel when others listen to you?
- How might an instructor's poor listening techniques affect the ability to teach students?
- How might good listening techniques affect an instructor's performance?

OVERVIEW

Section 2 focuses on developing effective listening skills and creating a supportive classroom environment. Student learning is enhanced when an instructor is engaged and understands what students may be saying—and not saying. Careful listening includes much more than hearing the question or the words spoken by a student.

Effective listening involves

- hearing and understanding students' questions or concerns and understanding what information they are seeking before you answer.
- paying attention to nonverbal communication.

- being sensitive to what is *not* being said.
- being aware of what message your listening style sends to the student.

Section 2 explores the components of effective listening. Attitudes and specific techniques are discussed in detail. Additionally, Section 2 points out specific ways that an instructor can help students develop their own effective listening skills for success, both in the classroom and in their careers. It also provides a basis for understanding student comments and motivations and guidelines for responding to student questions.

SUGGESTED GENERAL GUIDELINES: LISTENING TECHNIQUES

How important are effective listening skills to an instructor? How do you communicate the importance of listening to your students? What is your general assessment of your listening skills?

Assess your listening skills in each of the following areas. Under each heading, comment on your current practices related to the skill. For each, note your areas of strength as well as how you would like to improve. Use the information in the online component to guide your assessment and responses.

Develop a Willingness to Listen

Realize That You Are Not an Expert in Everything

Realize That You Cannot Read Your Students' Minds

Use Good Judgment When Bringing the Discussion Back to Yourself

Let Students Speak at Their Own Rate

Be Respectful of Other Perspectives

■ ■ ■ DIVERSITY CONSIDERATIONS ■ ■ ■

In some cultures, it is considered impolite to state needs directly. Develop an awareness of this as part of your listening skills so you can communicate more effectively with students from diverse backgrounds.

DIVERSITY REFLECTIONS

- What nonverbal messages might indicate that a student is having difficulty expressing his or her needs?

_____

_____

_____

_____

_____

- How can you help students express needs effectively in the Western workplace while respecting diverse backgrounds?

_____

_____

_____

_____

_____

Demonstrate That You Are Listening

Be Aware of Your Body Language

See the *Peer Review/Instructor Observation Form—Listening* at the end of this section.

REFLECTION QUESTIONS

Be sure to record your answers to these questions in the space provided and file them in the appropriate section of your Professional Development Portfolio.

- What other listening techniques have you seen to be effective? Ineffective?

_____

_____

_____

_____

_____

- What do you see as your listening strengths?

_____

_____

_____

_____

_____

- What areas would you like to improve?

_____

_____

_____

_____

_____

TEACHING STUDENTS HOW TO BE EFFECTIVE LISTENERS

What general strategies can you use to teach students effective listening skills? What strategies have you used in your classes?

Teach Students Specific Listening Techniques

What techniques can be taught in the classroom? Consider those summarized in the online content as well as other ideas that you have.

Ask Students to Apply Concepts of Active Listening in Class

What are the elements of active listening? How can you incorporate these into your classes?

Provide Students with the Skeletal Version of Your Outline

Consider providing a version of your outline to students. What is students' feedback? Record their input here.

Encourage Students to Paraphrase and Bullet Their Notes

Do your students re-write your words verbatim or do they paraphrase and record major points? How can you develop students' listening skills so they are able to paraphrase your lectures?

Give Students Permission to Disagree with Material Presented

How can giving students permission to disagree encourage listening skills? How do you encourage healthy disagreement and debate in your classes?

REFLECTION QUESTIONS

Be sure to record your answers to these questions in the space provided and file them in the appropriate section of your Professional Development Portfolio.

- How else do you teach students effective listening skills?

_____

_____

_____

_____

_____

- What specific activities or approaches can you apply in your classes that would support the development of listening skills?

_____

_____

_____

_____

_____

- What benefits will you gain in your classroom if students learn and consistently practice effective listening skills?

_____

_____

_____

_____

_____

- How did (or how could) active listening techniques affect the quality and outcome of the communication? (Review some of the interactions that you have had recently in your class or pay special attention to those that arise in the near future. Review the interactions and note where active listening techniques were applied, as well as where they could have been improved upon.)

_____

_____

_____

_____

_____

UNDERSTANDING STUDENT MOTIVATIONS

In what ways are motivation and listening related in your classes? What examples in the online component have you observed in your classes?

For each of the following categories, consider students that you have had in class. Do any students illustrate the needs discussed in the online course? Consider how you addressed each situation and evaluate if you could have done anything differently based on the information in the online course.

The Student Who Needs a Lot of Clarification

DIVERSITY CONSIDERATIONS

Be aware of situations in which a need for clarification is due to a special need or cultural difference. In these cases, work with the students to determine the most effective approach for them.

DIVERSITY REFLECTIONS

- What are some indications that a constant need for clarification might be due to a disability or other special need?

_____

_____

_____

_____

_____

- How would you approach a student in this situation?

_____

_____

_____

_____

_____

The Student Who Wants to Be Heard

The Student Who Wants to Confront the Instructor

The Student Who Does Not Participate

The Student with Low Self-Esteem

REFLECTION QUESTIONS

Be sure to record your answers to these questions in the space provided and file them in the appropriate section of your Professional Development Portfolio.

- List questions your students have asked which have an underlying motive. How did you respond?

_____

_____

_____

_____

- Was your response effective or ineffective? Why? (Brainstorm responses that may have achieved better results. It may be beneficial to complete this exercise with other instructors.)

_____

_____

_____

_____

_____

IMPLEMENTING EFFECTIVE LISTENING: GUIDELINES FOR HEARING AND RESPONDING TO STUDENT QUESTIONS AND COMMENTS

How effectively do you address students' questions and comments? How effectively do you respond to the negative situations outlined in the online component of the course?

For each of the following headings from the online course, assess how effectively you meet the criteria. Consider the suggested strategies in the course and note how you might use each to enhance your effectiveness in listening and responding to students' questions.

Be Genuinely Open to Questions

Set Time Aside for Questions and Use This Time

Respect All Responses

Make Sure You Understand the Question Before Answering It

Look Students in the Eye When They Respond

Listen to the Student's Complete Response

Schedule the Order of Your Responses

Repeat the Question So Everyone Can Hear

Admit When You Don't Know the Answer

Praise Students at Any Opportunity

REFLECTION QUESTIONS

Be sure to record your answers to these questions in the space provided and file them in the appropriate section of your Professional Development Portfolio.

- How do you praise students in your class? How often?

_____

_____

_____

_____

_____

- Describe a recent incident in which you were praised. How did you feel?

_____

_____

_____

_____

_____

- How might you develop your methods for providing positive reinforcement to students for their efforts in the classroom?

_____

_____

_____

_____

_____

Answer Most Questions Directly

Help Students Answer Their Own Questions

Make Sure Your Answer Is Accurate

Correct Wrong Answers

REFLECTION QUESTIONS

Be sure to record your answers to these questions in the space provided and file them in the appropriate section of your Professional Development Portfolio.

- What are two circumstances in which you successfully corrected wrong answers?

_____

_____

_____

_____

_____

- What are two circumstances you have observed in which students were corrected ineffectively? (Describe the differences in the two situations.)

_____

_____

_____

_____

_____

- How could elements from the successful situation be applied to the less successful one?

_____

_____

_____

_____

_____

- How can you apply this in your own classes?

_____

_____

_____

_____

_____

Respond to the Entire Class

Be Professional with Difficult Students

Control the "Know-It-All"

REFLECTION QUESTIONS

Be sure to record your answers to these questions in the space provided and file them in the appropriate section of your Professional Development Portfolio.

- What techniques have you used to successfully control the class "know-it-all"?

_____

_____

_____

_____

_____

- What unsuccessful methods have you used or observed? (Describe the differences in the two situations.)

_____

_____

_____

_____

_____

- How can you apply this in your classes?

_____

_____

_____

_____

_____

Control the Heckler

REFLECTION QUESTIONS

Be sure to record your answers to these questions in the space provided and file them in the appropriate section of your Professional Development Portfolio.

- What techniques have you used to successfully control the class heckler?

_____

_____

_____

_____

_____

- What unsuccessful methods have you used or observed? (Describe the differences in the two situations.)

_____

_____

_____

_____

- How could elements from the successful situation be applied to the less successful one?

_____

_____

_____

_____

_____

- How can you apply this in your classes?

_____

_____

_____

_____

_____

Rephrase and Redirect Students to the Positive

Answer Questions That Are Beyond the Scope of the Course After Class

Thank Students for Their Questions

Thank Students for Their Feedback

Confirm That Students' Questions Were Answered Sufficiently

Encourage Student-to-Student Interaction

Never Punish Students

REFLECTION QUESTIONS

Be sure to record your answers to these questions in the space provided and file them in the appropriate section of your Professional Development Portfolio.

- What other considerations are important when responding to student questions?

_____

_____

_____

_____

_____

- What effective classroom techniques have you used or observed?

_____

_____

_____

_____

_____

_____

LEARNING ACTIVITIES

The following activities are designed to support you in applying the module concepts to your teaching activities. Use the "Notes for Planning This Activity" spaces to record your ideas and to note resources. Complete each activity and submit as directed by your campus faculty development director. File copies of your activities and any evaluation comments you receive in your Professional Development Portfolio.

Listening Skills Activity

Complete the *Listening Self-Checklist* at the end of this section.

Notes for Planning This Activity:

Response to Student Questions and Comments Activity

 Review the list of questions and comments provided and determine exactly what the student might be asking. Identify possible motivations and/or the unmet need the student may have. Describe an appropriate approach to responding to the student. Also describe an inappropriate or ineffective response. To apply this to your own students, consider keeping a similar log of your responses to comments and questions that come up in your classes.

Complete the *Question/Comment Responses Form* at the end of this section.

Notes for Planning This Activity:

Best Case Review

 Upon completing Section 2, identify a situation in which you feel you utilized outstanding listening and response techniques with a positive outcome. Write a reflection paper on the experience, including:

- background information about the student (please use fictitious name).
- a description of the situation.
- the listening techniques you used.
- the response you gave and why you chose this approach.
- the outcome of the situation.
- anything you would do differently next time and why.

Notes for Planning This Activity:

Listening Techniques Online

Conduct an Internet search using "listening" or "listening techniques" as your search term. Gather useful online resources and review them with other instructors in your program or department. Brainstorm ways to apply the techniques in the classroom and devise a checklist to monitor your progress.

Notes for Planning This Activity:

LEARNING OBJECTIVES REVISITED

Review the Learning Objectives for Section 2 and rate your level of achievement for each objective using the rating scale provided. Following your assessment, determine the steps you need to take to meet the objective effectively. For each objective on which you do not rate yourself as a 3, outline a plan of action that you will take to achieve the objective fully. Include a time frame for this plan. Review completed Learning Activities for specific areas in which you need further development. Include the assessment and goals that you write in your Professional Development Portfolio. You may wish to use the Instructor Improvement Plan to set goals to further work toward learning objectives.

1 = did not successfully achieve objective
2 = understand what is needed, but need more study or practice
3 = achieved learning objective thoroughly

	1	2	3
2. The instructor will demonstrate the ability to use effective listening techniques in a classroom setting, including demonstrating the ability to understand a question before answering it, making students feel respected and valued, and showing a willingness to listen sincerely.	☐	☐	☐
3. The instructor will demonstrate the ability to identify motives behind student questions and make appropriate responses to their concerns.	☐	☐	☐

STEPS TO ACHIEVE UNMET OBJECTIVES

Steps	Date
1. _____	_____
2. _____	_____
3. _____	_____
4. _____	_____

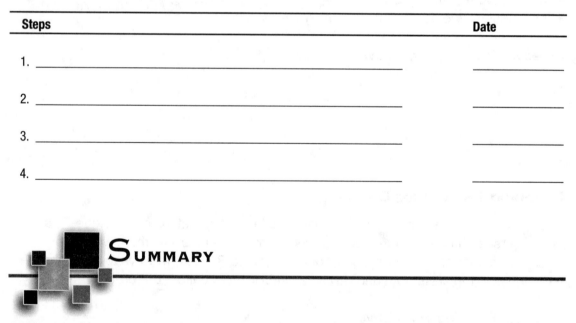

SUMMARY

Section 2 focused on developing effective listening skills and creating a supportive classroom environment. You were introduced to methods for ensuring that you truly understand students' questions before you answer. You also read about attitudes, specific listening techniques, and ways you can help students develop their own effective listening skills for success in the classroom and in their careers. You should now be able to describe and demonstrate effective listening techniques specifically for the college classroom setting. You should also be able to identify the motives behind student questions so the real needs of the students can be met.

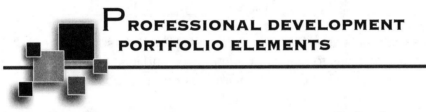

INSTRUCTOR IMPROVEMENT PLAN

Complete the Instructor Improvement Plan for Section 2 at this time. Take the necessary time to prepare a thoughtful, detailed improvement plan. Complete the form and keep it available as you plan and teach your classes for the next few terms. Note your progress, problems, successes, and questions over the next three to six months. At that time, reevaluate the plan and set new goals. Depending on the format you have selected for your Professional Development Portfolio, file the elements of your instructional plan in the appropriate sections. Record the dates for reassessing your goals on the professional development schedule at the beginning of your portfolio.

PROFESSIONAL DEVELOPMENT PORTFOLIO ELEMENTS

To finish Section 2, insert your completed responses, reflections, and activities from the section into the designated parts of your Professional Development Portfolio.

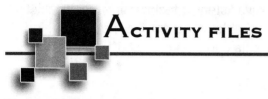

ACTIVITY FILES

The activities on the following pages will help you achieve the Section 2 learning objectives that are referenced throughout the section. In the online module, there are links to PDF files with supporting documents or worksheets for these activities.

PEER REVIEW/INSTRUCTOR OBSERVATION FORM—LISTENING

To the Instructor: Use this form for observation by a faculty member, your faculty training coordinator, or other professional colleague at your school. The focus of this review is on your listening skills during a classroom presentation. Remember to use any feedback that you receive in your Instructor Improvement Plan.

To the Reviewer: Please observe one of this instructor's classroom presentations and comment on the items listed below. Please be as specific as possible and give examples of behavior and actions whenever possible.

Date: _____ Class: _____

Comment on the instructor's general listening style and skills. Note such elements as willingness to listen, openness to different perspectives and ideas, and allowing the speaker to complete his or her thought. Feel free to add other observations as appropriate.

_____

_____

_____

_____

_____

_____

Comment on the instructor's use of self-disclosure. Consider factors such as amount of self-disclosure, timing, and appropriateness. Did the content of the self-disclosure add value to the presentation? Was there another approach that might have been more effective?

_____

_____

_____

_____

_____

_____

What did the instructor's body language communicate to the students? What demonstrated that the instructor was listening? What did not? Please be sure to give specific examples.

_____

_____

_____

_____

_____

_____

Please add any other comments or observations.

_____

_____

_____

_____

_____

_____

Please comment on strengths and make any suggestions for improvement that you feel would enhance this instructor's listening skills

_____

_____

_____

_____

_____

_____

LISTENING SELF-CHECKLIST

Instructions: Use this form to review your own listening techniques following a class you are teaching. Make an honest assessment of each item, noting any significant strengths or weaknesses you observe. Also, note any goals that you would like to add to your Instructor Improvement Plan. Be aware that, depending on the particular class, not all categories may apply. Consider printing additional copies and completing the checklist more than once to assess different areas or to assess your progress.

Date: _____ Class: _____

■ Demonstrated a willingness to listen.

_____

_____

_____

■ Used self-disclosure appropriately.

_____

_____

_____

■ Body language demonstrated openness to listening.

_____

_____

_____

■ Different perspectives were listened to, honored, and respected.

_____

_____

_____

■ Active listening techniques were discussed in class, or have been in the past.

_____

_____

_____

■ Students were encouraged to use active listening techniques.

_____

_____

_____

■ Students were assisted in developing effective listening skills for the purpose of note-taking, such as receiving a skeletal outline of the lecture or being given tips on note-taking (bulleted lists, paraphrasing).

_____

_____

_____

■ A sincere effort was made to understand and appropriately support student motivation.

_____

_____

_____

■ Students demonstrating demanding or otherwise difficult behavior were listened to and heard effectively, with issues being addressed appropriately.

_____

_____

_____

■ Actions demonstrated a sincere investment in hearing students' questions and concerns.

_____

_____

_____

■ Questions were answered promptly and directly, or an alternative session was set.

_____

_____

_____

■ All responses to questions posed in class were honored and respected.

_____

_____

_____

■ Student questions and comments were satisfactorily clarified.

_____

_____

_____

■ When several students volunteered to answer a question or comment on an issue, students were called on in a methodical manner.

_____

_____

_____

■ Students were allowed to complete their contribution without interruption.

_____

_____

_____

■ Students were appropriately reinforced for their contributions.

_____

_____

_____

■ Questions were answered directly, or students were encouraged to problem-solve, when appropriate.

_____

_____

_____

■ Answers were checked for accuracy and corrected as needed.

_____

_____

_____

■ Difficult students were handled in an appropriate manner.

_____

_____

_____

QUESTION/COMMENT RESPONSES

Instructions: Review the questions and comments below that could hypothetically be asked by a student. Use the information in the body of Section 2 to help you identify the context of the comment or situation. Consider that this is practice for when you will need to do the same in the classroom. For each comment or situation listed below:

- Identify possible motivations and/or the unmet need the student may have (if applicable).
- Describe an appropriate response or approach to the student.
- Describe an inappropriate or ineffective response or approach to the student.

To apply this to your own students, consider keeping a similar log of your responses to comments and questions that come up in your classes.

For practicing in a small group, separate scenarios on the lines between each example and distribute them for role-play and discussion.

Comment: *"You know, that information is really outdated."*

Possible Motivation or Need:

_____

_____

_____

Appropriate Response/Approach:

_____

_____

_____

Inappropriate Response/Approach:

_____

_____

_____

Comment: *"What do you mean by that? I still don't understand."*

Possible Motivation or Need:

_____

_____

_____

Appropriate Response/Approach:

_____

_____

_____

Inappropriate Response/Approach:

_____

_____

_____

Comment: *"Why would you say something like that? You know it's probably not true."*

Possible Motivation or Need:

_____

_____

_____

Appropriate Response/Approach:

_____

_____

_____

Inappropriate Response/Approach:

_____

_____

_____

Comment: *"I can probably never do well in this class. I'm the first one in my family to go to college and I have so many other responsibilities at work and at home."*

Possible Motivation or Need:

_____

_____

_____

Appropriate Response/Approach:

_____

_____

_____

Inappropriate Response/Approach:

_____

_____

_____

Situation: *A student presents a unique and unusual way of looking at an issue. It is very different and creative, yet practical and realistic.*

Possible Motivation or Need:

_____

_____

_____

Appropriate Response/Approach:

_____

_____

_____

Inappropriate Response/Approach:

_____

_____

_____

Comment: *"My aunt had a computer problem like that. We took it to three stores before anyone could figure out the problem. . . . Anyway, we thought it was a hard drive problem, but it wasn't. It turned out to be _____."*

Possible Motivation or Need:

_____

_____

_____

Appropriate Response/Approach:

_____

_____

_____

Inappropriate Response/Approach:

_____

_____

_____

Comment: *"World War II ended in 1950."*

Possible Motivation or Need:

_____

_____

_____

Appropriate Response/Approach:

_____

_____

_____

Inappropriate Response/Approach:

_____

_____

_____

Comment: *"I am just really skeptical about all this. The job market is so bad. I keep hearing there are no jobs in this field."*

Possible Motivation or Need:

_____

_____

_____

Appropriate Response/Approach:

_____

_____

_____

Inappropriate Response/Approach:

_____

_____

_____

Comment: *"Let me tell you about the healthcare insurance industry. The business people had to take it over. It was losing too much money. I don't care what anyone says—this system will mean better business in the long run. I know because I have lots of friends in the business." (And this goes on and on and on. . . .)*

Possible Motivation or Need:

_____

_____

_____

Appropriate Response/Approach:

_____

_____

_____

Inappropriate Response/Approach:

_____

_____

_____

Comment: *"I really think you lecture too much and that we need more visual aids and activities."*

Possible Motivation or Need:

_____

_____

_____

Appropriate Response/Approach:

_____

_____

_____

Inappropriate Response/Approach:

_____

_____

_____

SECTION

3

EFFECTIVE QUESTIONING TECHNIQUES

LEARNING OBJECTIVES

Upon successful completion of Section 3, the instructor will have achieved the following objectives. Check off each of the objectives as you have mastered it. You will have the opportunity to assess your performance on each objective at the end of Section 3.

4. The instructor will demonstrate the ability to identify various types of questions and when the different types can be used effectively in the classroom.
5. The instructor will demonstrate the ability to form strategic questions that encourage students to use higher levels of cognitive learning.

INTRODUCTORY QUESTIONS

- What kinds of questions can an instructor ask in class?
- Why is it important to use different forms of questions in class?
- How can you use questioning to develop critical thinking skills in students?

OVERVIEW

Section 3 outlines various forms of questions and discusses the ways instructors can use questions to facilitate learning in the classroom. It discusses how instructors can tailor questions to elicit higher-level thinking in students. It explores ways to respond to students' input in ways that encourage critical thinking and problem solving.

SUGGESTED GENERAL GUIDELINES: QUESTIONING TECHNIQUES

Review the findings regarding questioning techniques listed in the online course. Consider circumstances in your classes that illustrate these points. If you have made additional observations, add these to your comments.

TYPES OF QUESTIONS

What types of questions do you typically ask in your classes? Do you alter the types of questions you ask, and if so, how do you choose the type of question?

For each of the question types below, write an example question that you could use in one of your classes. Use the information provided in the online material to guide your question formulation.

Factual

Challenge

Application

Interpretation

Problem

Relational

Leading

Rhetorical

Critical

Diagnostic

Cause-and-Effect

Comparative

Hypothetical

Evaluative

Summation

Open-Ended Versus Closed-Ended

See the *Question Brainstorming Worksheet* at the end of this section.

REFLECTION QUESTIONS

Be sure to record your answers to these questions in the space provided and file them in the appropriate section of your Professional Development Portfolio.

- What other types of questions do you use successfully in your teaching?

_____

_____

_____

_____

_____

- What types of questions have you not thought of using? In what ways could they be effective in your class?

_____

_____

_____

_____

_____

_____

PREPARING QUESTIONS FOR VARIOUS COGNITIVE SKILL LEVELS

How aware are you of the different levels of questioning? How proficient are you at formulating questions based on the level of complexity at which students are expected to learn?

For each of the following headings, review the corresponding information in the online material. Define and write a sample question for each level of Bloom's taxonomy.

Knowledge

Comprehension

Application

Analysis

Synthesis

Evaluation

See the *Effective Questioning: Applying Bloom's Taxonomy* form at the end of this section.

REFLECTION QUESTIONS

Be sure to record your answers to these questions in the space provided and file them in the appropriate section of your Professional Development Portfolio.

- How often do you use different types of questions? (In the courses you teach, estimate the percentage of use for each of the following types of questions. Then, keep a tally of the types of actual questions you ask in your next three class sessions.)

Knowledge   _____

Comprehension   _____

Application   _____

Analysis   _____

Synthesis   _____

Evaluation   _____

_____

_____

_____

_____

_____

QUESTIONING TECHNIQUES

Record your ideas for developing effective questions. Consider strategies that you currently use.

As you complete the following sections of the online module, consider how you might develop additional strategies or improve on the ones that you use.

Plan Your Questions Ahead of Time

How do you currently incorporate questions into your lesson plans? Based on the suggestions in the online material, how can you do this more effectively?

Prepare Your Strategies for Asking Questions

How do you decide the format in which your questions will be asked and answered? How might you change your planning strategy based on the online material?

Determine the Purpose for the Question

How do you choose your questions? How can you make your questions more directed at a purpose?

Share the Purpose of Your Questions with Students

How do you make your students aware of the purpose of the questions you ask? How does increasing students' awareness improve their focus and critical thinking skills?

Train Students to Effectively Respond to Questions Early in the Class

How do you emphasize the importance of critical thinking and problem solving starting from the first day of class? How do you use questioning to accomplish this? How can you develop your use of questions to increase emphasis on these skills?

Solicit Questions from Students

How much do you emphasize students' ability to develop effective questioning skills? How do you encourage questioning at the higher levels of Bloom's taxonomy?

REFLECTION QUESTIONS

Be sure to record your answers to these questions in the space provided and file them in the appropriate section of your Professional Development Portfolio.

- What techniques do you use to help students formulate effective questions?

_____

_____

_____

_____

_____

- How might you improve this process in your classes?

_____

_____

_____

_____

- How effective do you find these techniques? (Apply a technique and write a brief review on its effectiveness, including what was successful, what was not, and ways in which you might alter the process to best fit your class situation.)

_____

_____

_____

_____

_____

Think Twice Before Asking, "Are There Any Questions?"

How effectively do you respond to students' questions?

Don't Put Students in the Hot Seat

Consider the suggestions provided in the online material and assess your questioning based on these criteria. Do you keep students "on their toes," or do they end up in the "hot seat?" How might you adjust your strategy?

Respect the Needs of Shy Students

How do you currently address the needs of shy students? How might you improve your responses to shy students based on the online course?

Rephrase Difficult Questions as Personal Curiosity Rather than Fact Seeking

How effectively do you phrase questions as curiosity or solution finding?

REFLECTION QUESTIONS

Be sure to record your answers to these questions in the space provided and file them in the appropriate section of your Professional Development Portfolio.

- Where might these techniques have been helpful in your most recent classes and lectures? How would you have worded your questions? What would the responses have been?

_____

_____

_____

_____

_____

- How might you use these techniques in upcoming classes and lectures?

  (Identify points in those lectures where this approach to questioning might be beneficial. Jot down possible questions in your lecture notes and try using them in class. After the class, reflect on the experience. What went well? What would you change? How would you improve the process?)

_____

_____

_____

_____

_____

Put the Student's Name at the *End* of the Question

Where do you insert the student's name when asking questions? What other techniques do you use for keeping the entire class engaged?

Maximize Questions

List some techniques you use to build on questions and to encourage student interaction using questions. Record additional ideas for developing these techniques.

Guide the Discussion with Your Questions

How do you currently use questions to guide discussion? How can you use questions as described in the online course to develop your discussion-guiding skills?

Ask Questions That Allow Students to Show You They Understand the Content

Provide an example of a time when you used questioning to determine students' understanding of the material. What was successful? What could have been improved upon, and how would you have improved the process?

Give Students Time to Answer

How long do you wait for students to respond to a question? Based on the online information, how would you change your approach?

Ask One Question at a Time

How well do you organize your questions? Consider how effectively students follow your questioning sequence. Based on the information in the online course, is there anything you would do to change how you organize your questions?

Ask Specific Questions Rather than Very Broad Questions

How well do you structure your questions? Consider how effectively your questioning sequence guides students to the point. Based on the information in the online course, is there anything you would do to change how you structure your questions?

For Complex Topics, Ask Questions That Do Not Rely on Complete Comprehension

Give an example of a question that you recently asked in class that was intended to encourage students to provide a complex response. How effective were you in reaching your goal? Assess whether your question was worded to elicit facts or encourage deeper thought. What changes could you make?

[   ]

Let Students Know if There is No Correct or Single Answer

How frequently do you ask questions that have no "right" answer? What are students' responses to these types of questions?

[   ]

REFLECTION QUESTIONS

Be sure to record your answers to these questions in the space provided and file them in the appropriate section of your Professional Development Portfolio.

- How have you presented questions with more than one correct answer in your classes?

  _____

  _____

  _____

  _____

  _____

- What are your observations when you use this technique?
  (Use this approach in your classes and write a short summary about your observations of students' responses.)

  _____

  _____

  _____

  _____

  _____

Seek Consensus and Opposing Viewpoints

How do you help students to consider additional viewpoints? Consider a time in class when you built consensus. How successful were you? What would you do differently?

■ ■ ■ DIVERSITY CONSIDERATIONS ■ ■ ■

Students from certain cultural backgrounds may consider disagreeing—especially with an authority figure such as a teacher—disrespectful. Respect the students' beliefs while encouraging discussion. If appropriate, discuss the situation with the students privately.

DIVERSITY REFLECTIONS

• How would you differentiate a lack of assertiveness from cultural influences?

_____

_____

_____

_____

_____

• How would you respectfully address this issue with a student?

_____

_____

_____

_____

_____

REFLECTION QUESTIONS

Be sure to record your answers to these questions in the space provided and file them in the appropriate section of your Professional Development Portfolio.

- What methods have you used in your classes to explore opposing points of view and to build consensus?

_____

_____

_____

_____

_____

- How can you expand these skills?

_____

_____

_____

_____

_____

Consider How You Ask Questions and How You Respond

What attitude do you convey to the class with your nonverbal communication? What feedback have you received regarding your nonverbal communication?

Use Physical Proximity to Facilitate Questioning

How do you use your physical position in the classroom to facilitate questioning? Based on the ideas in the online course, how might you use physical positioning as way to guide your class questions and discussion?

Praise Correct Responses

How consistently do you acknowledge correct responses? How do you ensure sincerity?

Note Questions for Future Reference

Do you currently keep a question log? Consider how doing so could contribute to the development of future courses.

LEARNING ACTIVITIES

The following activities are designed to support you in applying the module concepts to your teaching activities. Use the "Notes for Planning This Activity" spaces to record your ideas and to note resources. Complete each activity and submit as directed by your campus faculty development director. File copies of your activities and any evaluation comments you receive in your Professional Development Portfolio.

Peer Review: Questioning Techniques

Ask your faculty development coordinator, another instructor in your department, or other colleague at your school to observe you in class and to assess your questioning techniques. Provide them with the Peer Review/Instructor Observation Form for Questioning to use as a guide. Review and discuss your feedback and use the information in your Instructor Improvement Plan.

See the *Peer Review/Instructor Observation Form—Questioning* at the end of this section.

Notes for Planning This Activity:

Self-Assessment: Questioning Techniques

Using the Self-Review Form for Questioning, assess your questioning techniques in class. Note whether you use a certain technique and make notes regarding the technique's effectiveness, what you would change, students' reactions, and other observations. Make several copies of the form so you can make consecutive assessments and track your progress. You may also wish to compare your self-assessment results with those of your peer assessment and discuss the outcomes.

See the *Self-Review—Questioning* form at the end of this section.

Notes for Planning This Activity:

LEARNING OBJECTIVES REVISITED

Review the Learning Objectives for Section 3 and rate your level of achievement for each objective using the rating scale provided. Following your assessment, determine the steps you need to take to meet the objective effectively. For each objective on which you do not rate yourself as a 3, outline a plan of action that you will take to achieve the objective fully. Include a time frame for this plan. Review completed Learning Activities for specific areas in which you need further development. Include the assessment and goals that you write in your Professional Development Portfolio. You may wish to use the Instructor Improvement Plan to set goals to further work toward learning objectives.

1 = did not successfully achieve objective
2 = understand what is needed, but need more study or practice
3 = achieved learning objective thoroughly

	1	2	3
4. The instructor will demonstrate the ability to identify various types of questions and when the different types can be used effectively in the classroom.	☐	☐	☐
5. The instructor will demonstrate the ability to form strategic questions that encourage students to use higher levels of cognitive learning.	☐	☐	☐

STEPS TO ACHIEVE UNMET OBJECTIVES

Steps	Date
1. _____	_____
2. _____	_____
3. _____	_____
4. _____	_____

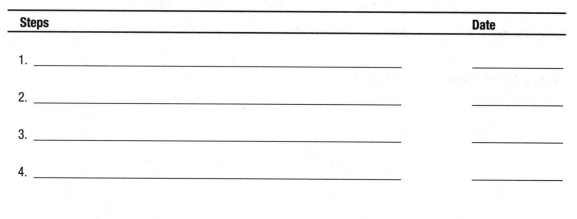

SUMMARY

Section 3 focused on developing techniques for using effective questioning to facilitate learning. You read about types of questions, the role each type plays in class dialogue, and how each is most effectively used. You also learned about Bloom's taxonomy and its relationship to questioning and the development of thinking skills. You should now be able to use questioning to facilitate discussion and create a positive learning environment.

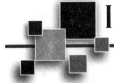

INSTRUCTOR IMPROVEMENT PLAN

Complete the Instructor Improvement Plan for Section 3 at this time. Take the necessary time to prepare a thoughtful, detailed improvement plan. Complete the form and keep it available as you plan and teach your classes for the next few terms. Note your progress, problems, successes, and questions over the next three to six months. At that time, reevaluate the plan and set new goals. Depending on the format you have selected for your Professional Development Portfolio, file the elements of your instructional plan in the appropriate sections. Record the dates for reassessing your goals on the professional development schedule at the beginning of your portfolio.

PROFESSIONAL DEVELOPMENT PORTFOLIO ELEMENTS

To finish Section 3, insert your completed responses, reflections, and activities from the section into the designated parts of your Professional Development Portfolio.

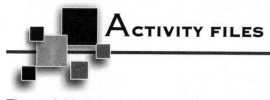

ACTIVITY FILES

The activities on the following pages will help you achieve the Section 3 learning objectives that are referenced throughout the section. In the online module, there are links to PDF files with supporting documents or worksheets for these activities.

QUESTION BRAINSTORMING

Instructions: For one of the classes you are teaching or will be teaching, list the main topics of the class in the left-hand column. In the right-hand column, list questions that you could pose to students that would support them in achieving the level of understanding suggested by your course objectives. Refer to "Types of Questions" in Module 3, Section 3 for guidelines. Make additional copies of this form as needed.

Topics   Possible Questions

_____   _____

_____   _____

_____   _____

_____   _____

_____   _____

_____   _____

_____   _____

_____   _____

_____   _____

EFFECTIVE QUESTIONING: APPLYING BLOOM'S TAXONOMY

By teaching students to consider information on a variety of levels, you help them become aware of different ways of thinking.

Instructions: Use this form to plan questions that can be used to encourage students to think at the different levels of the taxonomy as they apply to your topic of discussion. Based on your discussion topic, identify questions that relate to different levels. Some areas may not apply to your topic. Feel free to omit those that are not relevant, as well as to add others that are. Use these questions to guide your discussion in class. Remember to explain the levels of thinking to students and assist them in the process of self-questioning. Encourage them to engage in the processes of metacognition and to think about their thinking.

After the class in which you use this technique, complete the self-evaluation form following the questions.

Topic: _____

Knowledge

Ask students to:

■ **Identify reasons for an event.**
Sample questions for this topic:

_____

_____

_____

_____

■ **List characteristics or facts about an object, event, or process.**
Sample questions for this topic:

_____

_____

_____

_____

■ **Define terms and vocabulary.**
Sample questions for this topic:

_____

_____

_____

_____

■ **Recall information from reading or other sources.**
Sample questions for this topic:

_____

_____

_____

_____

In Summary: At the knowledge level, students should be able to demonstrate a clear understanding of the basic facts and information which provide the foundation of the topic at hand.

Comprehension

Ask students to:

■ **Discuss the reasons for a particular fact or event.**
Sample questions for this topic:

_____

_____

_____

_____

■ **Interpret information about a fact or event.**
Sample questions for this topic:

_____

_____

_____

_____

■ **Associate events based on their similarities and other characteristics.**
Sample questions for this topic:

_____

_____

_____

_____

■ **Describe consequences and outcomes based on the knowledge one has about a particular object or event.**
Sample questions for this topic:

_____

_____

_____

_____

■ **Make a reasonable calculation or estimation based on the knowledge they have.**
Sample questions for this topic:

_____

_____

_____

_____

In Summary: At the comprehension level, students should begin to demonstrate a deeper understanding of the material by applying it in familiar situations. Understanding is demonstrated within the same context that the information was learned. It is not necessarily applied to new situations.

Application

Ask students to:

■ **Use theoretical information to solve new problems.**
Sample questions for this topic:

_____

_____

_____

_____

■ **Use information to seek additional knowledge.**
Sample questions for this topic:

_____

_____

_____

_____

■ **Classify and modify information as appropriate to the situation.**
Sample questions for this topic:

_____

_____

_____

_____

■ **Provide an illustration or demonstration based on the knowledge that they have.**
Sample questions for this topic:

_____

_____

_____

_____

In Summary: At the application level of knowledge, students can use knowledge in practical, applied situations as well as use the information to problem solve. Information is applied to new situations, in addition to familiar ones.

Analysis

Ask students to:

■ **Understand the components of a problem or situation, as well as the components of its solution.**
Sample questions for this topic:

_____

_____

_____

_____

■ **Recognize and use patterns that are observed in various phenomena.**
Sample questions for this topic:

_____

_____

_____

_____

■ **Imply meanings from information that is presented or known.**
Sample questions for this topic:

_____

_____

_____

_____

■ **Compare and contrast theories, ideas, and other phenomena.**
Sample questions for this topic:

_____

_____

_____

_____

In Summary: At the analysis level of thinking, students can begin to break down what they know about a topic, see similarities and differences, and decipher meanings that are not obvious. Essentially, at the analysis stage, students are able to consider information in a more critical fashion.

Synthesis

Ask students to:

■ **Generalize information to new situations.**
Sample questions for this topic:

_____

_____

_____

■ **Generate ideas to add to an existing body of knowledge.**
Sample questions for this topic:

_____

_____

_____

_____

■ **Create new ideas and solutions.**
Sample questions for this topic:

_____

_____

_____

_____

■ **Bring related knowledge from different areas together.**
Sample questions for this topic:

_____

_____

_____

_____

In Summary: At the synthesis level of thinking, students are able to offer new ideas and solutions from existing knowledge. They are able to provide reasonable hypotheses based on known information and can integrate information from various sources into a coherent whole.

Evaluation

Ask students to:
■ **Compare and contrast different theories, ideas, premises, or actions.**
Sample questions for this topic:

_____

_____

_____

_____

■ **Adhere to one side of an argument and provide their rationale for doing so.**
Sample questions for this topic:

_____

_____

_____

■ **Assess the viability of information.**

Sample questions for this topic:

_____

_____

_____

_____

■ **Differentiate opinion from fact.**

Sample questions for this topic:

_____

_____

_____

_____

In Summary: At the evaluation stage of thinking, students are making judgments about information in terms of its accuracy, appropriateness for a situation, and its general viability.

Self-Evaluation Form—Self-Dialogue—Bloom's Taxonomy

What was your response to using this technique? Did you like it? Not like it? Why or why not?

_____

_____

_____

_____

How did the students respond?

_____

_____

_____

_____

How did the technique affect the class dynamic and activity? What was effective? What was not?

_____

_____

_____

_____

What would you change next time?

_____

_____

_____

_____

What else can you do to continue to reinforce this skill in future activities?

_____

_____

_____

_____

PEER REVIEW/INSTRUCTOR OBSERVATION FORM—QUESTIONING

To the Instructor: Use this form for observation by a faculty member, your faculty training coordinator, or other professional colleague at your school. The focus of this review is on your questioning skills during a classroom presentation. Remember to use any feedback that you receive in your Instructor Improvement Plan.

To the Reviewer: Please observe this instructor's use of questioning in a classroom presentation. Complete this feedback form by checking off, in the left-hand column, behaviors that you note during the presentation. In the right-hand column, please make any comments that you feel would be helpful. Please provide both positive and constructive feedback and be as specific as possible in your examples of behavior.

Date: _____ Class: _____

Instructor: _____

■ The instructor used a variety of question types.

_____

_____

_____

■ The instructor used questions that encouraged thinking and responses from a variety of cognitive levels.

_____

_____

_____

■ Questions seemed well-planned and prepared.

_____

_____

_____

■ The instructor shared the purpose and focus of questions with students.

_____

_____

_____

- The instructor encouraged students to develop their own questioning skills.

  _____

  _____

  _____

- The instructor's questioning technique was respectful of students' individual levels of comfort. The instructor avoided putting anyone on the "hot seat."

  _____

  _____

  _____

- The instructor used questioning as a way to guide the discussion and encourage interaction between students.

  _____

  _____

  _____

- The instructor used questions in a manner that promoted the development of information and discussion themes.

  _____

  _____

  _____

- The instructor asked questions in a manner that allowed students to show what they know.

  _____

  _____

  _____

- The instructor gave students ample time to answer the question before moving on to the next person or topic.

  _____

  _____

  _____

- Questions were posed one at a time.

  _____

  _____

  _____

- The instructor encouraged multiple viewpoints by letting students know if a question had no one correct answer.

  _____

  _____

  _____

■ The instructor tried to build consensus while honoring different viewpoints.

_____

_____

_____

■ The instructor encouraged participation with positive feedback, appropriate tone of voice, and nonverbal communication.

_____

_____

_____

SELF-REVIEW—QUESTIONING

To the Instructor: Use this form to review the questioning techniques you used during a given class. The categories to be reviewed correspond to the techniques discussed in Module 3, Section 3. It may be helpful, when using this form, to review the categories before your class.

When reviewing your class, comment on
- what you did to make questioning effective.
- how students responded.
- what went well.
- any changes you would like to make.

Use copies of this form to complete subsequent reviews and to track the development of your questioning techniques.

Date: _____ Class: _____

■ Questions reflected a variety of question types.

_____

_____

_____

_____

■ Questions encouraged thinking and responses from a variety of cognitive levels.

_____

_____

_____

_____

■ Questions were well planned and prepared.

_____

_____

_____

_____

■ The purpose and focus of questions were explained to students.

_____

_____

_____

_____

■ Students were encouraged to develop their own questioning skills.

_____

_____

_____

_____

■ Questions posed were respectful of students' individual levels of comfort. No one was put on the spot.

_____

_____

_____

_____

■ Questions guided the discussion and encouraged interaction between students.

_____

_____

_____

_____

■ Questions posed promoted the development of information and discussion themes.

_____

_____

_____

_____

■ The questions that were asked allowed students to show what they know.

_____

_____

_____

_____

■ The students had ample time to answer each question before the class moved on to the next person or topic.

_____

_____

_____

_____

■ Questions were posed one at a time.

_____

_____

_____

_____

■ Expression of diverse viewpoints was encouraged by letting students know if a question had no single correct answer.

_____

_____

_____

_____

■ Building consensus and honoring diverse viewpoints were priorities and were encouraged with questions.

_____

_____

_____

_____

■ Participation was encouraged with positive feedback, appropriate tone of voice, and nonverbal communication.

_____

_____

_____

_____

APPLIED QUESTIONING: LECTURE DEVELOPMENT ACTIVITY

Use the "Question Brainstorming" and "Effective Questioning: Applying Bloom's Taxonomy" activities completed previously in this section as a guide for this final activity. For a course you are or will be teaching, use your lesson plans to develop a set of questions that includes a wide variety of different question types. Insert them into your lesson plans at the appropriate points. It is acceptable to use some of the questions from the previous activity, but be certain they are appropriate to the topic and level of learning. Briefly state the purpose for using each question and what you want the students to learn. Include a minimum of 10 different question types.

Notes for Planning This Activity:

SECTION

4

EFFECTIVE LECTURE TECHNIQUES

LEARNING OBJECTIVES

Upon successful completion of Section 4, the instructor will have achieved the following objectives. Check off each of the objectives as you have mastered it. You will have the opportunity to assess your performance on each objective at the end of Section 4.

   6. The instructor will demonstrate the ability to develop an effective and interesting lecture for a college class.

INTRODUCTORY QUESTIONS

- What percent of your own teaching is lecture?
- When should a lecture be used? What kinds of information are best supported by lecture?
- What makes a lecture interesting and effective?
- What makes a lecture boring and ineffective?

OVERVIEW

Section 4 discusses effective lecture techniques that instructors of adult learners can use in the college classroom. Though lecture should not be the dominating teaching methodology for the adult learner, it is an effective delivery method for specific types of content. Section 4 discusses strategies for planning, giving, and following up on the dynamic and effective lectures that are appropriate for the adult learner.

SUGGESTED GENERAL GUIDELINES: CLASSROOM LECTURE TECHNIQUES

How effective are your lectures? Do they repeat information in the textbook? Are your lectures motivating to students? Review the general guidelines provided in the online course and make a general assessment of your lectures based on the criteria listed in the guidelines.

PURPOSES OF A LECTURE

For what purposes do you use lecture in your classes? How do you decide whether to use lecture or another teaching strategy?

Provide Current Material

How do you use lecture to update information from the textbook?

Organize Information for Students

Provide an example of how you have used lecture to organize course material for students. Refer to the examples of ways to organize material as listed in the online course.

Summarize Large Amounts of Material

How have you used lecture to summarize information from diverse sources?

Make Information Applicable

Provide an example of a time when you used lecture to apply general information to your specific field.

Motivate Students

Provide an example of a time when you used lecture to motivate or excite students about a topic.

REFLECTION QUESTIONS

Be sure to record your answers to these questions in the space provided and file them in the appropriate section of your Professional Development Portfolio.

- When have students been genuinely excited and motivated in one of your lectures? What caused students to react with enthusiasm? What was your own level of enthusiasm and excitement about the topic? What did you do that contributed to the enthusiasm of the class?

_____

_____

_____

_____

_____

- When were students *not* enthusiastic and motivated in your class? What were the differences between this class and the class in which students were genuinely enthused? What contributed to their lack of enthusiasm?

_____

_____

_____

_____

_____

- How can you recreate an atmosphere of enthusiasm and motivation in other classes?

_____

_____

_____

_____

_____

Explore Concepts and Applications

Review the "sandwich" technique described in the online course. How do you currently use lectures to explore concepts and their applications?

[ ]

See the *Sandwich Technique Worksheet* at the end of this section.

REFLECTION QUESTIONS

Be sure to record your answers to these questions in the space provided and file them in the appropriate section of your Professional Development Portfolio.

- What topics do you teach in your classes that would be effectively covered using the "Sandwich Technique"? (For a topic that you will be covering, plan a session using this method.)

_____

_____

_____

_____

_____

Model Behaviors and Processes

Think of a time when you wanted to demonstrate an abstract skill such as problem solving or logical thinking. How did you demonstrate it? How successful were you?

[ ]

REFLECTION QUESTIONS

Be sure to record your answers to these questions in the space provided and file them in the appropriate section of your Professional Development Portfolio.

- How do you demonstrate complex processes such as logical reasoning, problem-solving techniques, and decision-making strategies in your classes? (For a course that you are teaching or will be teaching, review your lesson plans and identify topics that require these thinking strategies.)

_____

_____

_____

_____

_____

- How can you demonstrate and describe these in your class? (Develop a plan using lecture to teach students the steps and skills that are involved.)

_____

_____

_____

_____

_____

Assess Student Progress

How do you currently use lecture to assess students' progress? How might you use it in the future?

REFLECTION QUESTIONS

Be sure to record your answers to these questions in the space provided and file them in the appropriate section of your Professional Development Portfolio.

- What topics that you currently teach (or that you plan to teach in the future) are ideal for lecture? (For each of the courses you are or will be teaching, list the specific topics that are best covered by lecture.)

_____

_____

_____

_____

_____

- What topics do you currently teach using lecture? How might they be more effectively covered using a different teaching methodology? (List these topics and write one or two alternative ideas for activities that would effectively cover these topics.)

_____

_____

_____

_____

_____

_____

PLANNING A LECTURE

How do you incorporate the four major considerations in planning a lecture into your class preparation? Provide examples from your course planning.

The Introduction

How do your introductions to lectures accomplish the goals of the introduction outlined in the online course? Provide an example from one of your lectures. Consider how well you have applied this to other classes.

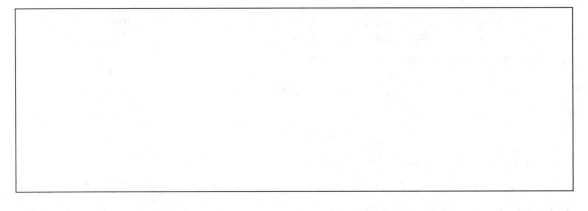

The Body

What is typically included in the bodies of your lectures? How do you incorporate other activities into the body? How successful are you? What would you like to improve?

The Conclusion

How effectively do your conclusions pull information together and accomplish the other goals outlined in the online module? How could you develop these additional goals in your classes?

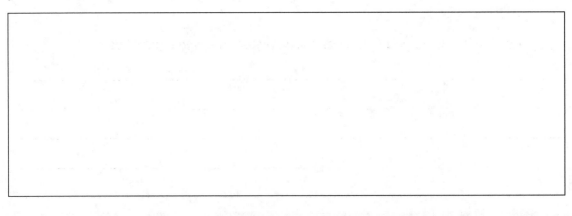

EFFECTIVE LECTURING TECHNIQUES

How do you balance the considerations listed in the online material? How do you meet diverse student needs within your classes?

Consider Students with Disabilities

What students do you currently have or have you had in the past who have a disability? Describe the accommodations you made for these students so that they could get the most from your lectures.

For each of the following types of disabilities, note accommodations that can be made in class to facilitate students' use of lecture in class. Note accommodations that have been successful for your students, those that have not, and note additional strategies that are not included in the online module.

■ ■ DIVERSITY CONSIDERATIONS ■ ■

When considering students with special needs, ask students what is most helpful to them. Many times, students with disabilities have defined what they need to succeed. Keeping communication lines open is a large part of effectively supporting students with special needs.

DIVERSITY REFLECTIONS

- How effectively do you communicate with students with disabilities?

_____

_____

_____

_____

_____

- How can you develop a process for identifying students who might be having difficulty?

_____

_____

_____

_____

_____

- What resources are available for these students on your campus?

_____

_____

_____

_____

_____

Hearing

Vision

Learning

Practice Excellent Presentation Techniques

What techniques do you use to plan your lectures? How successful are these techniques? How could you improve?

Look and Act Professional

Make an assessment of your professional presentation, both in and out of the classroom.

Clearly Explain How Your Lecture Is Organized

How do you typically organize the content of your lectures? How do you select an organizational strategy?

REFLECTION QUESTIONS

Be sure to record your answers to these questions in the space provided and file them in the appropriate section of your Professional Development Portfolio.

• How do you typically inform students about the organization of your lecture?

_____

_____

_____

_____

_____

• How do your students use your organization format to understand the material?

_____

_____

_____

_____

_____

_____

Limit Lecture Segments to 15 to 20 Minutes

What have you noticed about your students' attention spans during you lectures?

Limit Your Lecture to Three or Four Main Points

How many points are typically included in your lectures? How well do students digest the material provided in your lectures?

See the *Lecture Planning Sheet* at the end of this section.

REFLECTION QUESTIONS

Be sure to record your answers to these questions in the space provided and file them in the appropriate section of your Professional Development Portfolio.

- How long are your lecture segments? (Estimate the average length of the lectures of your classes. Then time your lecture chunks in your next five teaching sessions.)

_____

_____

_____

_____

_____

- Was your estimate accurate? Do you need to revise the length of your lectures? (Revise your lesson plan, adjust lecture segment length, and insert active learning techniques as needed to build the body of the lecture. Incorporate an effective introduction and conclusion.)

_____

_____

_____

_____

_____

_____

Begin and End the Lecture with a Summary

Where do you typically insert a summary into your lectures? Do you use summaries as effectively as possible? Why or why not?

Understand the Difference Between a Presentation and a Lecture

How do you differentiate between a lecture and a presentation? How can concepts of each be used in your classes?

REFLECTION QUESTIONS

Be sure to record your answers to these questions in the space provided and file them in the appropriate section of your Professional Development Portfolio.

- Are your lectures more reflective of a lecture or a presentation? (Review your lecture styles according to the criteria in the chart.)

_____

_____

_____

_____

_____

- What changes can you make to ensure your classroom presentations are meeting lecture criteria?

_____

_____

_____

_____

_____

Avoid Lecturing Strictly from Notes or a Script

Review the strategies for reducing reliance on notes or a script while lecturing. How can you apply these to develop your skills?

Find a Note Strategy That Works for You

What note strategy do you currently use? Which of the strategies listed in the online module do you currently use?

REFLECTION QUESTIONS

Be sure to record your answers to these questions in the space provided and file them in the appropriate section of your Professional Development Portfolio.

- What is the lecture note strategy that works best for you? Why is it effective? What about it is *not* effective?

_____

_____

_____

_____

_____

- Have you tried other strategies? Which strategies would you like to try? (For one of the classes that you are teaching or will be teaching consider using different note strategies that interest you and compare their styles.)

_____

_____

_____

_____

_____

Be Flexible in the Classroom

How aware are you of teachable moments in the classroom? How flexible are you in the classroom? How do you strike a balance between staying on track and remaining flexible? Consider examples from your teaching experience.

Let Students See the Real You

Provide an example of how you show your "real self" to students while maintaining appropriate professional boundaries. How would you like to develop this balance, and how can you accomplish this?

Move Around Your Classroom

How do you maintain contact with individual students in the midst of a large classroom situation? How does maintaining contact contribute to a successful class?

See the *Checklist for an Effective Lecture* at the end of this section.

REFLECTION QUESTIONS

Be sure to record your answers to these questions in the space provided and file them in the appropriate section of your Professional Development Portfolio.

- What techniques do you use to make your lectures effective? What do you see when you review the finished product? Do you fulfill your lecture plans? (Assess your lecture planning and actual delivery.)

_____

_____

_____

_____

_____

_____

EXPANDING THE LECTURE

How do you expand your lectures to involve students outside of the classroom?

Let Your Students Know You Are Teaching Each of Them as Individuals

How do you demonstrate respect for students as individuals? Have you used any of the strategies listed in the online module? Which ones (or others that you can think of) would be most effective with your students?

Offer a Variety of Ways to Reinforce Lecture Outside of Class

Which of the strategies for reinforcing lecture would be appropriate for your students and situation?

REFLECTION QUESTIONS

Be sure to record your answers to these questions in the space provided and file them in the appropriate section of your Professional Development Portfolio.

- What are some ways you currently make yourself available to students outside of class? What other methods would you like to try?

_____

_____

_____

_____

_____

- How does making yourself more available to students affect your relationship with them and the learning environment in your class? How have students responded to your efforts to help them outside of class? (Note any differences between students' responses when you provide quality extra assistance and when you do not. Reflect also on differences in your own attitude toward teaching and students.)

_____

_____

_____

_____

_____

Pay Attention to the Struggling Student

When have some of the "warning signs" listed in the online module indicated a struggling student in one of your classes?

REFLECTION QUESTIONS

Be sure to record your answers to these questions in the space provided and file them in the appropriate section of your Professional Development Portfolio.

- How do you help students who are having difficulty in your classes?

_____

_____

_____

_____

_____

- What additional methods could you use that would be effective in your specific courses?

_____

_____

_____

_____

_____

Pay Attention to the Most Successful Student in the Class

When have you noticed successful students in your class? How has their success influenced their performance in your class and school in general?

REFLECTION QUESTIONS

Be sure to record your answers to these questions in the space provided and file them in the appropriate section of your Professional Development Portfolio.

- How do you help the advanced students in your classes? What additional methods would be effective in your specific courses?

_____

_____

_____

_____

_____

Monitor Student Progress Continually in Class

How might you implement some of the activities for monitoring student progress suggested in the online module?

REFLECTION QUESTIONS

Be sure to record your answers to these questions in the space provided and file them in the appropriate section of your Professional Development Portfolio.

- How do you monitor student progress in your class (not including formal evaluation tools)?

_____

_____

_____

_____

_____

- What other methods would you like to try? (Implement one of the techniques described here and write a brief reflection on what you learned about yourself, your teaching, and students in the assessment process.)

_____

_____

_____

_____

_____

LEARNING ACTIVITIES

The following activities are designed to support you in applying the module concepts to your teaching activities. Use the "Notes for Planning This Activity" spaces to record your ideas and to note resources. Complete each activity and submit as directed by your campus faculty development director. File copies of your activities and any evaluation comments you receive in your Professional Development Portfolio.

Lecture Assessment

Either using a lecture you have presented in the past or a lecture presented by a colleague in a college course, use your Lecture Planning Worksheet to evaluate the different elements of the lecture. Make recommendations for improvement. Complete this evaluation in groups of three or four instructors who teach in similar areas.

Notes for Planning This Activity:

Lecture Development Activity

Using the Lecture Planning Worksheet for a course you are or will be teaching, develop a topical lecture using the techniques discussed in Section 4.

Notes for Planning This Activity:

LEARNING OBJECTIVES REVISITED

Review the Learning Objectives for Section 4 and rate your level of achievement for each objective using the rating scale provided. Following your assessment, determine the steps you need to take to meet the objective effectively. For each objective on which you do not rate yourself as a 3, outline a plan of action that you will take to achieve the objective fully. Include a time frame for this plan. Review completed Learning Activities for specific areas in which you need further development. Include the assessment and goals that you write in your Professional Development Portfolio. You may wish to use the Instructor Improvement Plan to set goals to further work toward learning objectives.

1 = did not successfully achieve objective
2 = understand what is needed, but need more study or practice
3 = achieved learning objective thoroughly

	1	2	3
6. The instructor will demonstrate the ability to develop an effective and interesting lecture for a college class.	☐	☐	☐

STEPS TO ACHIEVE UNMET OBJECTIVES

Steps	Date
1. _____	_____
2. _____	_____
3. _____	_____
4. _____	_____

SUMMARY

Section 4 focused on planning and developing an effective lecture for the adult learner. You read about specific guidelines and techniques instructors can use to deliver a lecture effectively. You also leaned about a lecture's purpose, strategies for planning lectures, effective techniques for lectures, and methods for expanding lectures beyond the classroom. You should now be able to use these techniques along with the presentation skills described in Section 4, while noting the differences between presentations and lectures.

INSTRUCTOR IMPROVEMENT PLAN

Complete the Instructor Improvement Plan for Section 4 at this time. Take the necessary time to prepare a thoughtful, detailed improvement plan. Complete the form and keep it available as you plan and teach your classes for the next few terms. Note your progress, problems, successes, and questions over the next three to six months. At that time, reevaluate the plan and set new goals. Depending on the format you have selected for your Professional Development Portfolio, file the elements of your instructional plan in the appropriate sections. Record the dates for reassessing your goals on the professional development schedule at the beginning of your portfolio.

PROFESSIONAL DEVELOPMENT PORTFOLIO ELEMENTS

To finish Section 4, insert your completed responses, reflections, and activities from the section into the designated parts of your Professional Development Portfolio.

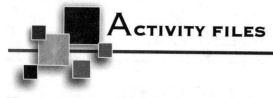

ACTIVITY FILES

The activities on the following pages will help you achieve the Section 4 learning objectives that are referenced throughout the section. In the online module, there are links to PDF files with supporting documents or worksheets for these activities.

SANDWICH TECHNIQUE

Instructions: Select one of your topics and corresponding course objectives that would be effectively taught using the "Sandwich Technique." Use this document to plan the three elements of the method.

Topic: _____

Course Objectives:

_____

_____

_____

_____

_____

Background Information

Reading Assignments:

_____

_____

_____

_____

Web Sites:

_____

_____

_____

_____

Other Resources:

_____

_____

_____

_____

Major Points of Focus:

_____

_____

_____

_____

Lecture

Address Students' Questions:

_____

_____

_____

_____

Review of Major Points of Focus:

_____

_____

_____

_____

Applications of Concepts:

_____

_____

_____

_____

Real-World Examples:

_____

_____

_____

_____

Other Information:

_____

_____

_____

_____

Activity

Goal:

_____

_____

_____

Select as many formats as applicable:

❏ Whole class ❏ Computer lab

❏ Small group ❏ Field trip

❏ Pairs ❏ Demonstration

❏ Individual ❏ Research/Presentation

❏ In-class ❏ Other_____

❏ Homework

Time Frame:_____

Materials:

_____

_____

_____

_____

Instructions:

_____

_____

_____

_____

Major Points of Follow-up Discussion:

_____

_____

_____

_____

LECTURE PLANNING WORKSHEET

Instructions: Use this sheet to plan segments of your lecture and insert active learning techniques between lecture components. Practice incorporating elements of the introduction, body, and conclusion where indicated. Depending on your topic and the length of your session, you may need fewer or more sections. Adjust this form to meet your needs. Once the lecture is planned, use it in class. Actively review the process and note what worked well for you and what did not. Use this activity to plan the capstone project for Section 4 of Module 3.

Topic: _____

Course Objectives Covered in This Session:

_____

_____

_____

_____

_____

Introduction

Overview of Topic and Objectives:

_____

_____

_____

_____

_____

Relationship to Earlier Material:

_____

_____

_____

_____

_____

Thought-Provoking Questions:

_____

_____

_____

_____

_____

Organization of Lecture:

_____

_____

_____

_____

_____

Body

Lecture Segment 1

Main Points:

_____

_____

_____

_____

_____

Techniques (Discussion, Questions, Analogies, Examples, etc.):

_____

_____

_____

_____

_____

Relationship to Past and Future Learning:

_____

_____

_____

_____

_____

Active Learning 1

Activity Description, Format, and Materials:

_____

_____

_____

_____

_____

Instructions:

_____

_____

_____

_____

_____

Follow-Up:

_____

_____

_____

_____

_____

Lecture Segment 2

Main Points:

_____

_____

_____

_____

_____

Techniques (Discussion, Questions, Analogies, Examples, etc.):

_____

_____

_____

_____

_____

Relationship to Past and Future Learning:

_____

_____

_____

_____

_____

Active Learning 2

Activity Description, Format, and Materials:

_____

_____

_____

_____

Instructions:

_____

_____

_____

_____

_____

Follow-Up:

_____

_____

_____

_____

_____

Lecture Segment 3

Main Points:

_____

_____

_____

_____

_____

Techniques (Discussion, Questions, Analogies, Examples, etc.):

_____

_____

_____

_____

_____

Relationship to Past and Future Learning:

_____

_____

_____

_____

_____

Active Learning 3

Activity Description, Format, and Materials:

_____

_____

_____

_____

_____

Instructions:

_____

_____

_____

_____

_____

Follow-Up:

_____

_____

_____

_____

_____

Conclusion

Review of Main Points:

_____

_____

_____

_____

_____

Relevance of Session to Career and Workplace:

_____

_____

_____

_____

_____

Questions or Method of Student Assessment:

_____

_____

_____

_____

_____

Final Summary and Lead-In to Next Class:

_____

_____

_____

_____

_____

CHECKLIST FOR AN EFFECTIVE LECTURE

To the Instructor: This checklist can be used in a variety of ways. Use it to

- assess a lecture before you deliver it. Review your plan for a specific class to see that you have considered all the important elements of the lecture.
- review your delivery of a lecture. If an element was not adequately covered, assess what was lacking and make necessary changes in your preparation.
- pursue an ongoing professional development goal. Complete the assessment and review processes on a continuing basis. Record your observations and progress in a learning journal.

Some of the items in the checklist may apply to both the assessment and review process. Use those that are appropriate to the process you are using. For items with an is/was or are/were choice, consider the item in present tense for the assessment process and in past tense for the review process. For assessment, assess whether the element is planned for in lesson plans and notes. For the review, assess whether the element was effectively covered and conveyed in the class.

❑ Lecturer develops or has a plan to develop rapport with students.

❑ Lecturer captures or has a method to develop students' attention at beginning.

❑ Lecturer holds or has a plan to effectively hold students' attention.

❑ Content is accurate.

❑ Content is/was appropriate for level of student.

❑ Content is relevant to the course in general.

❑ Content directly addresses or supports learning objectives of the class.

❑ Structure of lecture is/was understandable and clearly stated.

❑ Lecturer did not read from text or notes nor recite from memory.

❑ Key points are/were emphasized and made obvious.

❑ Concepts are/were explained clearly.

❏ Concepts are/were explained in two or three different ways.

❏ Examples are/were used.

❏ Lecturer refers or referred to previous lecture or content.

❏ Lecturer refers or referred to future lecture or content.

❏ Lecturer refers or referred to text and other supporting tools available to students.

❏ Lecturer plans to address or did address homework assignments, activities, labs, or other learning activities.

❏ Voice was clear.

❏ All students could hear.

❏ Visual aids and other resources are planned to be used or were used to supplement the presentation.

❏ Visual aids were easily seen and read.

❏ Cues were given to students to assist them in taking notes.

❏ Pace of presentation was appropriate.

❏ Lecturer made eye contact appropriately with each student.

❏ Lecturer has plans to include or did include active learning.

❏ Opportunity for asking questions is/was provided.

❏ Lecturer listened to student questions.

❏ Lecturer responded to questions effectively and positively.

❏ Lecturer encouraged further learning outside of classroom.

❏ Lecturer was enthusiastic.

❏ The conclusion of the lecture summarized the main points.

❏ Lecturer was interesting to the students.

❏ Lecture content is/was applied to field(s) of study.

CUSTOMIZED LECTURE PLANNING WORKSHEET

Develop a worksheet that you can use to plan the lectures for your course. Complete this activity in groups of three to five instructors. Use the Lecture Planning Worksheet created earlier in Section 4. Develop the sheet using additional considerations, including planning techniques, effective delivery techniques, and ways to expand beyond the lecture itself. Make it specific to the courses you teach.

Notes for Planning This Activity:

SECTION

5

EFFECTIVE DISCUSSION TECHNIQUES

LEARNING OBJECTIVES

Upon successful completion of Section 5, the instructor will have achieved the following objectives. Check off each of the objectives as you have mastered it. You will have the opportunity to assess your performance on each objective at the end of Section 5.

7. The instructor will demonstrate the ability to begin, facilitate, and summarize an interesting discussion.
8. The instructor will demonstrate the ability to recognize and overcome barriers to discussion and list ways to gain the participation of all students using the various techniques discussed.
9. The instructor will demonstrate the ability to develop and implement a minimum of five different discussion activities for use in a current or future course. The instructor will then evaluate the effectiveness of the discussion activity and provide ways to enhance or revise the technique.

INTRODUCTORY QUESTIONS

- How much time do you spend in discussion in your classes on average? Monitor the discussion time in the next five class sessions you teach. Do you think that your discussion time is appropriate?
- What are the benefits of using discussion in the classroom with adult learners?
- How do the group dynamics in your class affect discussion?
- What are some problems or barriers to using discussion in the classroom with adult learners?

OVERVIEW

Section 5 covers effective discussion techniques, focusing on facilitation techniques and group process. It emphasizes the educational benefits of discussion in the learning process and provides practical strategies and activity suggestions for encouraging and improving discussion among adult learners.

SUGGESTED GENERAL GUIDELINES: EFFECTIVE DISCUSSION TECHNIQUES

How would discussion complement your lectures? How can discussion help your students develop professional and interaction skills?

Purposes of Discussion

What other purposes for discussion can you think of? How effectively do you currently plan class discussions?

REFLECTION QUESTIONS

Be sure to record your answers to these questions in the space provided and file them in the appropriate section of your Professional Development Portfolio.

- Where in your current classes would discussion be an effective learning tool?

_____

_____

_____

_____

_____

- What are some topics in your classes that could be effectively explored through structured discussion?

_____

_____

_____

_____

_____

BENEFITS OF DISCUSSION

What examples of effective discussion have you observed in your classes? Record examples of benefits to students that you have noticed.

REFLECTION QUESTIONS

Be sure to record your answers to these questions in the space provided and file them in the appropriate section of your Professional Development Portfolio.

- What other benefits of discussion can you think of that are important to the adult learner?

_____

_____

_____

_____

_____

TEACHING STUDENTS TO DISCUSS

List elements and ideas from Module 3 that you believe will be important for teaching students effective discussion skills.

REFLECTION QUESTIONS

Be sure to record your answers to these questions in the space provided and file them in the appropriate section of your Professional Development Portfolio.

- How can techniques for engaging students in lecture and questioning be applied to discussion?

_____

_____

_____

_____

_____

Tell Students Your Expectations About Discussion

Record the expectations that you will set for participation in discussion.

Emphasize the Benefits of Discussion

List the benefits of discussion that you will emphasize to students.

Set Discussion Guidelines

Which of the guidelines listed in the online module would you recommend for your classes? How will you involve students in setting the guidelines for discussion?

REFLECTION QUESTIONS

Be sure to record your answers to these questions in the space provided and file them in the appropriate section of your Professional Development Portfolio.

- What ground rules or guidelines for discussion have you established in your classroom?

_____

_____

_____

_____

_____

- How effective are they?

_____

_____

_____

_____

_____

- Based on the lists above, what would you add or delete? How can you involve students in this process?

_____

_____

_____

_____

_____

Teach Students General Discussion Strategies

Select strategies from the list provided online. Note methods for incorporating these strategies into your classes.

■ ■ ■ DIVERSITY CONSIDERATIONS ■ ■ ■

Help students to be aware of effective discussion techniques when working in a group that includes someone with a hearing impairment. Teach students to sit in a position that allows lip reading. Other techniques include using handouts when possible, repeating questions and comments, and summarizing main points.

DIVERSITY REFLECTIONS

- What other techniques might be useful for a student with a hearing impairment?

_____

_____

_____

_____

_____

- In a case of severe hearing impairment, what resources are available for a signer?

_____

_____

_____

_____

_____

REFLECTION QUESTIONS

Be sure to record your answers to these questions in the space provided and file them in the appropriate section of your Professional Development Portfolio.

- What other methods could you use to prepare your students for class discussions? (Implement these methods and record the effects on the discussion. Consider making notes in your lesson plans to indicate where you can use these techniques.)

_____

_____

_____

_____

_____

Start Small, Then Move Toward More Difficult Discussions

How will you introduce students to discussion concepts and strategies? What would be a good topic to start with? How will you increase expectations?

Organize the Discussion

To what topic might you apply the steps outlined in the online module? Consider creating a sample outline of your topic using these four steps.

REFLECTION QUESTIONS

Be sure to record your answers to these questions in the space provided and file them in the appropriate section of your Professional Development Portfolio.

- What other methods could you use to help organize discussions?

_____

_____

_____

_____

_____

- Where would these methods be most effective in your classes? (Consider researching discussion techniques and sharing them in your program or department.)

_____

_____

_____

_____

_____

Model Good Problem-Solving Techniques

Make note of the problem-solving techniques listed in the online module. Which would be effective in your classes? Identify topics or activities that would be effectively supported by these techniques.

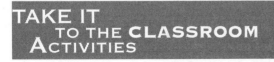

Take It to the Classroom activities are designed to support you in applying the module's concepts to the classroom. Course objectives will be met most effectively and learning will be most beneficial if the activities are completed in conjunction with the material found in the online course.

The following techniques can help students become effective problem solvers in classroom discussions. In the space provided for activity planning, note how you can incorporate these concepts into your classroom discussions. Note that some may be more appropriate than others for certain topics. (See Module 7: Teaching Students How to Learn for additional techniques and more detailed discussion of some techniques.)

Brainstorming

In brainstorming, a group offers ideas in a spontaneous manner. The goal is to generate as many ideas or solutions to a problem as possible. Quantity is the goal, and all ideas—including outrageous ones—are welcome and recorded for consideration. Write ideas on the board or a flip chart so everyone can see. (The visual part is important.) Some of the basic rules of brainstorming are to not pass judgment on any ideas during the generation period, to record all ideas, and to require participation by everyone in the group. When the generation phase is complete, review and evaluate the ideas. Participants build on the ideas that have been presented to create new ones. Consider the outrageous ideas for their merits or other inspiration they might spark. Record the new ideas that occur.

Notes for Planning This Activity:

Alternative to Brainstorming

This alternative to traditional brainstorming starts with a brief explanation of the problem to be solved and an explanation of the process. For 10 minutes, ask students to generate ideas silently and write them on a piece of paper. At the end of that time, go around the room and record the idea each student considers his or her best idea. Any discussion at this time should be limited to clarification rather than judgment. If desired, go around the room and list the second best idea on the paper. When all the ideas have been posted, ask students to rank the top three to five ideas. Take a vote to reach consensus on the top three ideas. Use these ideas for discussion and for making a decision.

Notes for Planning This Activity:

Benchmarking

In benchmarking, students compare the process or system they develop with an established process or system developed by recognized experts. First, identify the processes to use as a standard to benchmark against. Second, identify the standard. Third, collect and analyze data and information. Next, for each category or area, compare the students' benchmark to the standard and determine if the students' process is above or below the standard. When all benchmarks or areas have been compared, the class can develop an improvement plan.

Notes for Planning This Activity:

Assumption Identification

It is important in discussions, especially when trying to solve a problem, to differentiate assumptions (ideas one believes to be true) from facts and to evaluate assumptions critically. Students are often not aware of their own assumptions or others' assumptions as they discuss or pose ideas. A deliberate effort to identify assumptions trains students to become more aware of the importance of doing this and makes them more effective communicators. Acknowledge that all people make assumptions and that assumptions serve purposes, such as speaking to an issue with purpose and reflecting values that underlie problem solving. Assumptions can also set limits to a problem and simplify issues so that a reasonable discussion can be conducted. The disadvantage of assumptions is that they can hinder creativity or block the problem-solving process. Encourage students to be aware of their own assumptions and assess their validity carefully, and to reconsider assumptions that are arbitrary or wrong.

To help students become aware of their assumptions, define *assumptions* and list several assumptions on the board. To help students identify their assumptions, suggest categories in which assumptions are commonly made, such as time, money or budget, cooperation with others, physics, legal issues, energy or effort, cost/benefit, information, or cultural issues. Students may list additional categories. Discuss how these assumptions may come about and talk about their effects.

To further examine assumptions, list limitations and constraints on the board. For each limitation, list any assumptions that contribute to the limitation. For each assumption, determine if that limitation is valid or if it should be reconsidered.

Notes for Planning This Activity:

Multiple Views of Problem Solving

Teach students to consider more than one problem-solving strategy. The most common strategy is to look at the problem, identify and evaluate alternative solutions, and choose a solution to solve the problem. Suggest sequencing the process differently to gain an alternative perspective. Teach students to start with the solution—or what they believe the solution should be—and work backwards. This process sometimes makes the solution obvious. Also, consider beginning the process somewhere in the middle and working toward either end. For example, if you are making widgets but do not have either the funding or the market, consider how you would make the widgets, then work backward to develop the funding plan while working forward to develop the market for your widgets. In certain circumstances, this approach is effective and efficient.

Notes for Planning This Activity:

Cause-and-Effect Diagrams

This technique visually diagrams a problem or effect, its potential causes, and their interrelationships. The first step is to identify the problem and major categories of potential causes. These should be written in diagram form on the board or on a flip chart. Next, the group brainstorms specific causes in each major category. The third step is to eliminate causes that do not apply and to document the reasons why. The group then discusses the remaining causes and prioritizes them into two categories: "easiest to fix" and "most significant." Finally, each cause is evaluated to determine if it should be eliminated, controlled or altered, or accepted.

Notes for Planning This Activity:

S.W.O.T. Analysis

"S.W.O.T." stands for "strengths, weaknesses, opportunities, and threats." A S.W.O.T. analysis is used to evaluate these four elements of a plan. The goal of a S.W.O.T. analysis is to recognize positive circumstances and potential problems related to a plan and revise the plan so it can be implemented with success. Some examples of commonly asked questions in the phases of a S.W.O.T. analysis are:

- Strengths. What are the advantages? What do the participants do well?
- Weaknesses. What needs to be improved? What is done poorly? What deficiencies do participants have? What are negative perceptions?

- Opportunities. What are the possibilities? Are there any advantageous environmental elements?
- Threats. What are the negative elements in the environment? What are the obstacles? What is the competition?

Notes for Planning This Activity:

Developing Multiple Hypotheses

When developing a hypothesis (a reasonable explanation about a causal relationship), teach students to develop more than one hypothesis. This technique teaches students to look for alternative causes, relationships, assumptions, and interpretations. Remind students about bias. Explain the difference between causation and correlation and explain some of the confounding variables that can affect conclusions. Advise students about the problems associated with emotional attachment to one theory, which may create bias and cause them to overlook other possibilities.

Notes for Planning This Activity:

Consensus Building

In consensus building, all participants agree on a decision after discussing the advantages and disadvantages of several alternatives. First, brainstorm ideas and record them on the board. Eliminate duplicate, inappropriate, and impossible alternatives, and combine elements of similar ideas. Students then select the two to five ideas they consider to be the best alternatives. Record these top ideas and list the advantages and disadvantages of each one. Based on the analysis, select the choice with the greatest impact. Check with each participant for individual support. Even if the option is not everyone's first choice, each participant should be able to support the decision.

Notes for Planning This Activity:

Multiple Voting

This process can be used to reduce a large list to a more manageable size. List all ideas, such as those from a brainstorming session, on the board. Move down the list and vote on each idea. Let each student vote on multiple items, but permit only one vote per item. After the first round of voting, erase items with the fewest votes. Select the ideas with the most votes or look for the natural breaking point. Take a second vote; this time, each student can vote for half of the remaining items. Continue the voting rounds until three to five options remain. Avoid voting down to only one item.

Notes for Planning This Activity:

Developing a Model

Models are representations of ideas or problems so that all factors, characteristics, and elements can be more clearly viewed and understood. Models can make a problem more concrete or show hidden relationships. They also can make a very complex problem simple in order to facilitate discussion.

Notes for Planning This Activity:

Metaphors

A metaphor is a specific type of model that can be used to stimulate ideas and discussion by comparing one thing to another. For example: How is this problem like a garden? Ideas can be generated with similar characteristics, such as growth, weeds, vegetables, fruits, trees, shrubs, seeds, pruning, fertilizer, drought, floods, pests, and so forth. How is this problem like a machine? Ideas can be generated with similar characteristics, such as parts working together, machine operators, operating instructions, maintenance, worn or faulty parts, grease, power, output, and so forth. Any number of metaphors can be used to generate ideas.

Notes for Planning This Activity:

Critical Analysis

Critical analysis involves examining ideas, processes, or projects for flaws, discrepancies, or omissions. Emphasize that analysis of this type is done in a constructive spirit and with the intention of objective evaluation. (Remind students that this differs from negativity.) One way to maintain a constructive atmosphere is to require students to substantiate any criticism they provide. For example, a student who refutes another student's suggestion should support the refutation with a statistic or some other relevant fact.

Equally important is teaching students how to receive constructive criticism and use it to improve an idea or project. Frequently, students have been conditioned to become defensive toward feedback and constructive criticism. One of the challenges is to change the perception that being critiqued is "bad." Establish the culture in your class that feedback is not intended as overt criticism, but is directed at improvement. Some suggestions for achieving this include:

- replacing the word "criticism" with "feedback" or "suggestion" or some other ego-saving word.
- conducting critical analysis in small groups rather than with the entire class until students are accustomed to being critiqued.
- teaching students to word criticism in positive and supportive statements that lead to improvement.
- asking students how they prefer to receive criticism and asking them to provide feedback to classmates using the same consideration. This skill will serve students well in the workplace.
- teaching students to ask for critique in positive ways that will generate positive responses.
- encouraging students to separate their personal identities from their ideas so that self-esteem is not damaged.

Tell your students that feedback from individuals with different experiences, backgrounds, and perspectives will enrich their learning by exposing them to different ways of thinking. Students will undoubtedly experience multiple points of view in the workplace. Start with positive experiences, and as students become accustomed to evaluation, encourage them to ask for analysis of weaknesses and faults.

Notes for Planning This Activity:

Force Analysis

In a force analysis, a plan or idea is represented in the center of a diagram. On the right, list the forces working for the plan. On the left, list the forces working against the plan or idea. This visual representation allows a clear comparison of the support and opposition for a plan or idea. This overview of the big picture facilitates discussion. By looking at the forces for and against the plan or idea, students can alter or eliminate the plan or the forces.

Next, score each force, using 1 to indicate weak and 5 to indicate strong. Total the force rating in each column. Alter or eliminate forces by changing the plan, and then re-calculate the force rating. After making all the changes, determine the viability of the project.

Notes for Planning This Activity:

Heuristic Methods

A heuristic is a guide or rule of thumb that is generally learned by trial and error or a "learn-as-you-go" type of strategy. It involves intuition or gut feelings rather than certainty. These types of guidelines can be useful in the problem-solving discussion if used in a systematic manner. Structure the heuristic method by keeping detailed records of trials and their results. Narrow the choices by discarding approaches that prove ineffective.

When selecting or guiding students toward a problem-solving approach in a discussion, consider factors such as the nature of the problem or question the class is discussing, individual personalities, and the overall skill level of the class. Some methods will be better suited for certain types of questions or issues. Select the approach that most efficiently addresses the goals for the discussion. For example, if the class is discussing the introduction of a management model, a S.W.O.T. analysis might provide greater insight than using metaphors.

Consider students' characteristics and abilities as well. Choose a method that will optimize their personalities and skills as well as avoid potential clashes. Consider the known personality differences that could potentially disrupt and hinder the discussion. Healthy disagreement is beneficial and is different from overt and disruptive clashes. Likewise, consider the ability level of students and the background they will need to successfully engage in the selected method. If necessary, alter the method or provide foundational information.

Notes for Planning This Activity:

See the *Discussion Activity Plan and Review* form at the end of this section.

REFLECTION QUESTIONS

Be sure to record your answers to these questions in the space provided and file them in the appropriate section of your Professional Development Portfolio.

- What other strategies have you used to teach students to discuss and problem solve effectively?

_____

_____

_____

_____

_____

- Which method is most effective for an upcoming discussion planned for your class?

_____

_____

_____

_____

_____

- How does this method address the objectives of the discussion?

_____

_____

_____

_____

_____

- Will you need to adapt the method to meet students' personalities and abilities? If yes, how?

_____

_____

_____

_____

_____

- Review the outcome of the discussion. What went well? What would you change?

_____

_____

_____

_____

_____

DISCUSSION TECHNIQUES

What techniques do you currently use to facilitate class discussions? What would you like to improve?

List All Words or Terms That May Be Unfamiliar

How familiar are students with terminology used in class discussion? How can you familiarize them with terminology?

Plan the Discussion

How do you currently plan class discussions? How could you improve your planning and how would this improve discussions?

Begin the Discussion Thoughtfully

Which of the strategies from the list provided online do you think would be effective in your classes? How might you use information from other sections of Module 3 to begin discussion effectively?

Facilitate the Discussion Effectively

Which of the techniques listed have you used in your class discussions? Which were effective? Why? Which ones were less effective? Why? How would you like to develop your facilitation skills?

Using Group Dynamics to Facilitate Discussion

How familiar are you with group dynamics? What methods from those discussed in the module have you used during discussions? How would you like to develop your knowledge of group dynamics in the classroom?

■ ■ DIVERSITY CONSIDERATIONS ■ ■ ■

Remember that cultural background can influence the way a student participates in group activities. Develop an understanding of diverse cultural norms for group participation and incorporate these respectfully into your classroom activities.

DIVERSITY REFLECTIONS

- What kinds of ground rules could you establish for group activities that would create a supportive environment for diverse participation styles?

_____

_____

_____

_____

- How can you learn more about culturally diverse participation styles?

_____

_____

_____

_____

_____

Role of the Instructor

What is your typical role during class discussion? How do you view your role as a facilitator?

Group Techniques

Which of the group techniques discussed in the online module have you used in class discussions? Make an assessment of how effectively you use them and how well they support your facilitation of the discussion. Note areas in which you would like to expand your skills.

See the _Group Dynamics Checklist_ at the end of this section.

REFLECTION QUESTIONS

Be sure to record your answers to these questions in the space provided and file them in the appropriate section of your Professional Development Portfolio.

- What are your observations about your own group discussion facilitation techniques?

_____

_____

_____

_____

_____

- Which techniques have you used? Which would you like to try?

_____

_____

_____

_____

_____

- What are your thoughts about using group dynamics?

_____

_____

_____

_____

_____

Provide Closure for the Discussion

Which of the closure techniques from the online material would be effective in your classes? Which have you tried? Which ones would you like to try?

Evaluate the Discussion

Which of the evaluation techniques would be effective in your classes? Which have you tried? Which ones would you like to try?

Use Online Discussion Forums

Have you ever tried online discussion? In what class would you like to try it? What are the steps for developing an online class component at your institution?

■ ■ ■ DIVERSITY CONSIDERATIONS ■ ■ ■

If you do incorporate online discussion into your classroom activities, be sure that accommodations are made for students with special needs so that the discussion is easily accessible to them.

DIVERSITY REFLECTIONS

- What types of modifications can be made for increasing accessibility to online discussion?

_____

_____

_____

_____

_____

- How can your information technology department assist you in learning more about these features on your online platform?

_____

_____

_____

_____

_____

BARRIERS TO DISCUSSION

What are some of the barriers to class discussion that you have experienced? How did you address them?

Students Who Will Not Participate

Review the recommendations for addressing students who will not participate. How have you addressed these students in the past? Which techniques might be helpful in the future?

■ ■ DIVERSITY CONSIDERATIONS ■ ■

Certain emotional disorders can result in reluctance to participate in group discussions and activities. Be aware of these situations and help students participate within their level of comfort.

DIVERSITY REFLECTIONS

- How does the Americans with Disabilities Act (ADA) support individuals with emotional disorders?

_____

_____

_____

_____

_____

- How can you support these students respectfully, effectively, and in a manner that shows consideration for their privacy?

_____

_____

_____

_____

_____

_____

Students Who Participate Too Much

Review the recommendations for addressing students who participate too much. How have you addressed these students in the past? Which techniques might be helpful in the future?

Students Who Are Not Prepared for Effective Discussion

Review the recommendations for addressing students who are not prepared. How have you addressed these students in the past? Which techniques might be helpful in the future?

Students Who Argue Rather than Discuss

Review the recommendations for addressing students who argue rather than discuss. How have you addressed these students in the past? Which techniques might be helpful in the future?

LEARNING ACTIVITIES

The following activities are designed to support you in applying the module concepts to your teaching activities. Use the "Notes for Planning This Activity" spaces to record your ideas and to note resources. Complete each activity and submit as directed by your campus faculty development director. File copies of your activities and any evaluation comments you receive in your Professional Development Portfolio.

Building Discussion Skills

Develop a critique sheet to evaluate a college instructor facilitating a discussion involving adult learners. Develop this form in groups of two or three instructors. Additionally, use this form to evaluate a colleague (or a video of yourself leading a discussion) and make detailed recommendations for improvement.

Notes for Planning This Activity:

Discussion Topic Development

Develop a minimum of five discussion activities for use in a course you are or will be teaching.

Notes for Planning This Activity:

Comprehensive Discussion Project

For a topic in your class, select one of the discussion activities you developed. Devise a basic plan applying general discussion and group process techniques that you select based on guiding the group towards its goals. Review the group process; note effective versus ineffective techniques. Set a plan to continue to assess and develop your group process skills.

Notes for Planning This Activity:

LEARNING OBJECTIVES REVISITED

Review the Learning Objectives for Section 5 and rate your level of achievement for each objective using the rating scale provided. Following your assessment, determine the steps you need to take to meet the objective effectively. For each objective on which you do not rate yourself as a 3, outline a plan of action that you will take to achieve the objective fully. Include a time frame for this plan. Review completed Learning Activities for specific areas in which you need further development. Include the assessment and goals that you write in your Professional Development Portfolio. You may wish to use the Instructor Improvement Plan to set goals to further work toward learning objectives.

1 = did not successfully achieve objective
2 = understand what is needed, but need more study or practice
3 = achieved learning objective thoroughly

	1	2	3
7. The instructor will demonstrate the ability to begin, facilitate, and summarize an interesting discussion	☐	☐	☐
8. The instructor will demonstrate the ability to recognize and overcome barriers to discussion and list ways to gain the participation of all students using the various techniques discussed.	☐	☐	☐
9. The instructor will demonstrate the ability to develop and implement a minimum of five different discussion activities for use in a current or future course. The instructor will then evaluate the effectiveness of the discussion activity and provide ways to enhance or revise the technique.	☐	☐	☐

STEPS TO ACHIEVE UNMET OBJECTIVES

Steps	Date
1. _____	_____
2. _____	_____
3. _____	_____
4. _____	_____

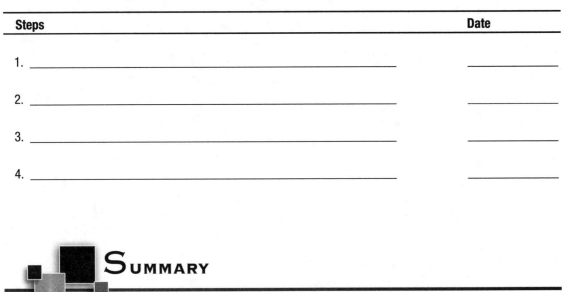

Summary

Section 5 covered effective discussion techniques, focusing on facilitating discussion and avoiding barriers to participation. You read about the educational benefits of discussion in the learning process and about techniques for in-class and online discussions. You learned about the application of group process and dynamics to classroom discussions. You should now be able to describe a variety of effective discussion techniques, develop a plan for teaching students how to participate in discussions, and create innovative discussion activities for your courses.

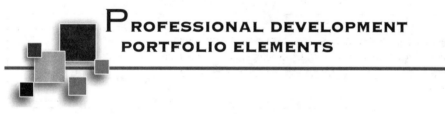

INSTRUCTOR IMPROVEMENT PLAN

Complete the Instructor Improvement Plan for Section 5 at this time. Take the necessary time to prepare a thoughtful, detailed improvement plan. Complete the form and keep it available as you plan and teach your classes for the next few terms. Note your progress, problems, successes, and questions over the next three to six months. At that time, reevaluate the plan and set new goals. Depending on the format you have selected for your Professional Development Portfolio, file the elements of your instructional plan in the appropriate sections. Record the dates for reassessing your goals on the professional development schedule at the beginning of your portfolio.

PROFESSIONAL DEVELOPMENT PORTFOLIO ELEMENTS

To finish Section 5, insert your completed responses, reflections, and activities from the section into the designated parts of your Professional Development Portfolio.

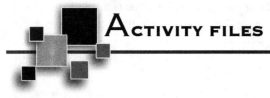

ACTIVITY FILES

The activities on the following pages will help you achieve the Section 5 learning objectives that are referenced throughout the section. In the online module, there are links to PDF files with supporting documents or worksheets for these activities.

DISCUSSION ACTIVITY PLAN AND REVIEW

Use this form to plan and review a discussion activity in one of your classes. Consider completing it for more than one activity and noting the development of discussion activities in your classes.

Date: _____ Class: _____

Topic: _____ Activity: _____

❑ List the objectives of the discussion.

_____

_____

_____

_____

_____

❑ Write a brief description of the discussion activity.

_____

_____

_____

_____

_____

❑ How does the activity meet the objectives of the discussion?

_____

_____

_____

_____

_____

❑ What personality characteristics and abilities need to be considered?

_____

_____

_____

_____

_____

❑ List any adaptations to be made to accommodate for personality or ability consider-ations. (For example, should certain people work or not work together? Is there any background information that should be provided to students before the activity?)

_____

_____

_____

_____

_____

❑ List major points or questions that you want to include in the discussion.

_____

_____

_____

_____

_____

❑ How will you implement ground rules for discussion and encourage students to use general discussion strategies?

_____

_____

_____

_____

_____

Review and Assessment

❑ How well did the activity meet the discussion objectives? What was successful?

_____

_____

_____

_____

_____

❑ What would you do differently?

_____

_____

_____

_____

_____

❑ How did individual personalities affect the discussion process? How effective were any adaptations that you made for personality or background knowledge?

_____

_____

_____

_____

_____

❑ How did you see students applying the ground rules for discussion that you set in the class? How did you encourage them to do so?

_____

_____

_____

_____

_____

❑ How did you see students using general strategies for discussion? How did you encourage them to do so?

_____

_____

_____

_____

_____

❑ What changes would you make based on your observations and students' responses during this discussion?

_____

_____

_____

_____

GROUP DYNAMICS CHECKLIST

The checklist that follows is intended to be used as a method of planning a strategy for facilitating group process in your class. For each group facilitation skill, assess how it might be used in an upcoming class discussion.

Following the activity, evaluate the group process using the evaluation form. Use the space to make observations and notes, and add other questions that you believe will enhance your understanding of the group process in your class. You can also use the checklist as a guide in class discussions and activities to help students understand and internalize the process involved in groups.

❑ What commonalities are shared between the class members? How might you use these relative to this topic?

_____

_____

_____

_____

_____

❑ What professional interaction skills can be expected in this activity? How might you identify them and encourage their use? How will you give feedback on their use?

_____

_____

_____

_____

❑ What types of interactional characteristics (for example, assertiveness, constructive criticism, confrontation, and others) might arise in this activity? How will these skills be evaluated and addressed in this activity? How can individual group members gain insight into their own interpersonal skills?

_____

_____

_____

_____

❑ How can the experiences and knowledge of individual group members be utilized in this group experience?

_____

_____

_____

_____

❑ What might come up in this activity that has the potential to cause individuals to examine their assumptions and beliefs? Is the topic controversial? How will conflict be addressed?

_____

_____

_____

_____

_____

❑ To accomplish the goals of the group, what skills (such as questioning, pointing out commonalities, gently confronting, and others) do you anticipate using? What would be the desired outcome of using the skills that you identify?

_____

_____

_____

_____

_____

Self-Evaluation Form—Group Dynamics

Use this form to evaluate the group dynamics within your class and your skills as a facilitator. For each of the items below, review the group process and the techniques that you used to facilitate it. Compare the results to the Group Dynamics Checklist that you completed before the class. Assess what went well and consider what you might change in order to improve the group process.

❑ What commonalities were shared between the class members? How did sharing affect the group process? What did you do to point out commonalities between class members?

_____

_____

_____

_____

_____

❑ What professional interaction skills were used in this activity? What did you do as facilitator to encourage their use? How did you give feedback on their use?

_____

_____

_____

_____

_____

❑ What types of interactional characteristics (for example, assertiveness, constructive criticism, confrontation, and others) were observed during the activity? How were these characteristics evaluated and addressed in this activity? How did individual group members gain insight into their own interpersonal skills?

_____

_____

_____

_____

_____

❑ How were the experiences and knowledge of individual group members utilized in this group experience?

_____

_____

_____

_____

_____

❑ What occurred in this activity that caused individuals to examine their assumptions and beliefs? Was the topic controversial? How was any conflict addressed?

_____

_____

_____

_____

_____

❑ To accomplish the goals of the group, what skills (such as questioning, pointing out commonalities, gently confronting, and others) did you use? What were the outcomes?

_____

_____

_____

_____

_____

❑ What would you do differently next time? What would you repeat?

_____

_____

_____

_____

_____

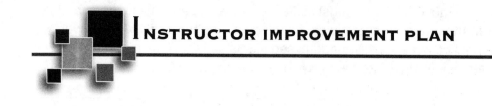

INSTRUCTOR IMPROVEMENT PLAN

Suggestions for Completing this Plan

1. Take the Premodule Assessment to determine your baseline knowledge of effective presentation skills.
2. Read the outline and note the objectives of the "Techniques for Classroom Presentation" module. Doing so will provide you with background information that will assist you in better assessing your skill level in this area.
3. List the questions you would like to find answers to or topics you want to explore in this section.
4. Use the information obtained from suggestions 1 through 3 above to complete this plan.

AREAS OF STRENGTH

Based on the information gathered by completing the Premodule Assessment, reviewing the objectives and outline, and composing your list of questions and topics, list your strongest presentation skills. These items should reflect things that you currently do in your classroom that you believe to be your strongest assets.

AREAS FOR DEVELOPMENT

Again, based on the information gathered by completing the recommended activities above, create a list of general areas in which you feel you could develop your classroom presentation skills. These should be general areas, such as "using visual aids" or "giving effective lectures." These general areas will be used to develop specific goals.

GOAL SETTING

A format in table form for setting goals and identifying resources can be found on the following page. One plan should be completed for each long-term goal that you establish. When writing your goals, the following guidelines are suggested:

1. Goals should be realistic and achievable. Considering your other life commitments, time availability, and other aspects of your particular situation, set goals that you can realistically achieve and that will provide you with a sense of accomplishment.

2. Write goals that are understandable. Be clear and concise. Your goals should be clearly stated so when you review them in the future, you can plainly understand the direction in which you planned to head. Likewise, a supervisor or colleague should also be able to clearly understand your intention when reading your goals.

3. Your goals should be measurable. In other words, there should be a concrete, observable product or behavior at the completion of each goal. When this product or behavior is satisfactory, you will know your goal has been achieved. Write your goals to reflect behavioral outcomes that you or another individual can observe.

4. Break your goals into long-term and short-term components. The long-term goal reflects the final outcome that you wish to achieve. The short-term component outlines the smaller elements that you will complete en route to completing the long-term goal. Short-term goals are helpful in gauging your progress toward completing your larger objective.

5. Review and revise goals regularly. Evaluate your goals and your progress periodically and on a regular basis. Goals can certainly be revised and revamped as your needs suggest. The Instructor Improvement Plan format provides an option for revisiting and revising your goals. A change to a goal does not mean failure.

6. Brainstorm sources of information that will provide you with resources for completing your goal. Resources can take many forms, including print material, electronic and audio-visual media, professional organizations, and supervisors or mentors, to name a few. Establish a general idea of where you wish to find information and investigate your possibilities. You may be surprised at the additional resources that present themselves as you complete this process.

INSTRUCTOR IMPROVEMENT PLAN

Name: _____ Date Developed: _____

| Long-Term Goal: | | | | | |
SHORT-TERM GOALS	METHOD AND RESOURCES FOR ACHIEVING GOAL	TARGET DATE FOR COMPLETION	DATE COMPLETED	OUTCOMES	REVISION/DATE

PROFESSIONAL DEVELOPMENT PORTFOLIO

PORTFOLIO ORGANIZATION SUGGESTIONS

I. Portfolio Part 1: Introduction

- Premodule Assessment*
- Initial Instructor Improvement Plan and Reflection*

II. Portfolio Part 2: Resource Development

(Include information that you print from the module or find in support of the learning activities.)

Section 1: Dynamic Presentation Techniques

Section 2: Effective Listening Techniques
- Listening Techniques Online Resources

Section 3: Effective Questioning Techniques

Section 4: Effective Lecture Techniques

Section 5: Effective Discussion Techniques

III. Portfolio Part 3: Practice and Development: Activities and Reflections

Section 1: Dynamic Presentation Techniques
- Reflection Questions (Complete the reflection questions diligently and add them to the portfolio. Some of your responses to reflection questions will provide examples and feedback that will complement other portfolio artifacts.)
- Physical Environment Checklist
- Attention Grabbers Brainstorming Worksheet
- Visual Aids Worksheet
- Lecture Planning Worksheet
- Lecture Assessment
- Lecture Development Activity

Section 2: Effective Listening Techniques
- Reflection Questions (Complete the reflection questions diligently and add them to the portfolio. Some of your responses to reflection questions will provide examples and feedback that will complement other portfolio artifacts.)

Section 3: Effective Questioning Techniques
- Reflection Questions (Complete the reflection questions diligently and add them to the portfolio. Some of your responses to reflection questions will provide examples and feedback that will complement other portfolio artifacts.)
- Question Brainstorming

- Effective Questioning: Applying Bloom's Taxonomy
- Applied Questioning: Lecture Development Activity

Section 4: Effective Lecture Techniques
- Reflection Questions (Complete the reflection questions diligently and add them to the portfolio. Some of your responses to reflection questions will provide examples and feedback that will complement other portfolio artifacts.)
- "Sandwich" Technique Worksheet
- Lecture Planning Practice Sheet

Section 5: Effective Discussion Techniques
- Discussion Activity Plan and Review
- Group Dynamics Checklist (Preparation Portion)
- Discussion Critique Form and Evaluation
- Discussion Activity Development

IV. Portfolio Part 4: Feedback

(Include information from your class evaluations and instructor observations.)

Section 1: Dynamic Presentation Techniques
- Faculty and Student Evaluations (Institution-Specific)
- Visual Aid Review
- Teaching Development Review

Section 2: Effective Listening Techniques
- Peer Review/Instructor Observation Form—Listening
- Listening Self-Checklist

Section 3: Effective Questioning Techniques
- Peer Review/Instructor Observation Form—Questioning
- Self Review—Questioning

Section 4: Effective Lecture Techniques
- Checklist for an Effective Lecture
- Lecture Assessment

Section 5: Effective Discussion Techniques
- Group Dynamics Checklist (Self-Evaluation Portion)
- Peer Review—Discussion Facilitation

V. Portfolio Part 5: Reassessment

- Postmodule Assessment*
- Continuing Instructor Improvement Plan and Reflection* **

VI. Portfolio Part 6: Capstone

Section 1: Dynamic Presentation Techniques
- Completed Lecture Planning Worksheet* **
- Completed Lecture Development Activity* **

Section 2: Effective Learning Techniques
- Question/Comment Responses* **

Section 3: Effective Questioning Techniques
- Applied Questioning: Lecture Development* **

Section 4: Effective Lecture Techniques
- Customized Lecture Planning Sheet* **
- Lecture Development Activity* **

Section 5: Effective Discussion Techniques
- Comprehensive Discussion Development Project* **

* Pull for Professional Development Documentation Portfolio
** Pull for Showcase Portfolio

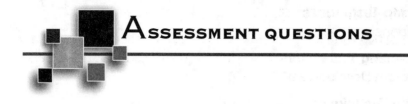

ASSESSMENT QUESTIONS

Section 1: Effective Presentation Techniques

1. Discuss the importance of the audience, the physical environment, the material, and the presenter to the success of a presentation.

2. What are the long-term positive effects of establishing rapport with students? Describe three methods for building rapport that would be effective for you and explain why these are appealing.

3. Select two methods for capturing and keeping students' attention that you believe to be effective. Briefly discuss why these would be effective with your students and source material.

4. Compare and contrast an effective visual aid with an ineffective visual aid. Please use examples. If possible, use examples of effective and ineffective visual aids that you have observed.

Section 2: Effective Listening Techniques

5. Section 2 focused on effective listening skills. Based on these concepts, select two skills and discuss how an instructor's ineffective listening techniques can adversely affect her or his ability to teach effectively.

6. How can instructors develop listening skills in students? Briefly discuss three techniques and suggest a method for implementing these in the classroom.

7. Explain the relationship between student motivation and effective listening.

Section 3: Effective Questioning Techniques

8. Discuss three benefits to students of asking various types of questions in class.

9. Describe five types of questions and describe how you would use each in your classes. Explain your rationale for selecting the questions you chose.

10. Identify a topic on which you would be likely to ask questions in one of your classes. Write one question that reflects each level of Bloom's taxonomy.

Section 4: Effective Lecture Techniques

11. Select two topics from a class you are currently teaching and discuss ways that lecture can be used appropriately to support them.

12. Consider the recommendations made in Section 4 for students with disabilities. Often, making these modifications to a classroom in a general way not only serves the needs of students with disabilities, but also enhances the environment for all students. Select two modifications from each of the subheadings (vision, hearing, and learning) and explain how you could implement them in your class.

Section 5: Effective Discussion Techniques

13. Select two topics from a class you are currently teaching and explain ways that discussion can be used appropriately to support them.

14. The benefits of discussion are overviewed in Section 5. Identify a time when you addressed a sensitive topic or had difficulty making a point in class. Explain how discussion might have improved the situation.

15. Select one of the strategies outlined in Section 5 for teaching students to use discussion. Select two strategies and describe how you would incorporate each into one of your classes.

16. Select one of the problem-solving methods listed in Section 4. Describe how you would use the technique in your class by applying it to a specific lesson plan.

17. Identify a group discussion or interaction in class that did not progress in ideal fashion. Discuss the group dynamics that occurred during the interaction. How did the dynamics affect the outcome of the discussion? How might they have been different? What could you have done to change the outcome?

18. Identify a situation in one of your classes that presented a barrier to discussion. Compare your handling of the situation to the techniques recommended in the module. Discuss what you would do the same in a similar situation as well as what you would do differently.

ASSESSMENT ANSWER KEY

The following are references to the answers for the Assessment Questions for Module 3. Information that serves as the basis for the answers in this section can be found in Sections 1-5. To make the information relevant to you, apply it thoughtfully to your individual situation.

Section 1: Effective Presentation Techniques

1. Discuss the importance of the audience, the physical environment, the material, and the presenter to the success of a presentation.

   Answer should make reference to the Delivery Techniques section of the module.

2. What are the long-term positive effects of establishing rapport with students? Describe three methods for building rapport that would be effective for you and explain why these are appealing.

   Answer should make reference to the Establishing Rapport with Students section of the module.

3. Select two methods for capturing and keeping students' attention that you believe to be effective. Briefly discuss why these would be effective with your students and source material.

   Answer should make reference to the following:
   - Capturing Students' Attention section
   - Keeping Students' Attention section

4. Compare and contrast an effective visual aid with an ineffective visual aid. Please use examples. If possible, use examples of effective and ineffective visual aids that you have observed.

   Answer should make reference to the Visual Aids section.

Section 2: Effective Listening Techniques

5. Section 2 focused on effective listening skills. Based on these concepts, select two skills and discuss how an instructor's ineffective listening techniques can adversely affect her or his ability to teach effectively.

   Answer should make reference to the following:
   - All sections can provide a basis for the answer to this question. Responses should compare effective listening techniques to ineffective ones and then compare the effects of each on students. Answers may vary depending on the instructor.

6. How can instructors develop listening skills in students? Briefly discuss three techniques and suggest a method for implementing these in the classroom.

   Answer should make reference to the Teaching Students How to Be Effective Listeners section.

7. Explain the relationship between student motivation and effective listening.

   Answer should make reference to the Understanding Student Motivation section.

Section 3: Effective Questioning Techniques

8. Discuss three benefits to students of asking various types of questions in class.

   Answer should make reference to the Suggested General Guidelines: Questioning Techniques section.

9. Describe five types of questions and describe how you would use each in your classes. Explain your rationale for selecting the questions you chose.

   Answer should make reference to the Types of Questions section.

10. Identify a topic on which you would be likely to ask questions in one of your classes. Write one question that reflects each level of Bloom's taxonomy.

    Answer should make reference to the Preparing Questions for Various Cognitive Skill Levels section.

Section 4: Effective Lecture Techniques

11. Select two topics from a class you are currently teaching and discuss ways that lecture can be used appropriately to support them.

    Answer should make reference to the Purposes of a Lecture section.

12. Consider the recommendations made in Section 4 for students with disabilities. Often, making these modifications to a classroom in a general way not only serves the needs of students with disabilities, but also enhances the environment for all students. Select two modifications from each of the subheadings (vision, hearing, and learning) and explain how you could implement them in your class.

    Answer should make reference to the Effective Lecturing Techniques section, Consider Students with Disabilities subheading.

Section 5: Effective Discussion Techniques

13. Select two topics from a class you are currently teaching and explain ways that discussion can be used appropriately to support them.

    Answer should make reference to the Purposes of Discussion section.

14. The benefits of discussion are overviewed in Section 5. Identify a time when you addressed a sensitive topic or had difficulty making a point in class. Explain how discussion might have improved the situation.

    Answer should make reference to the Benefits of Discussion section.

15. Select one of the strategies outlined in Section 5 for teaching students to use discussion. Select two strategies and describe how you would incorporate each into one of your classes.

    Answer should make reference to the Teaching Students to Discuss section, Teach Students General Discussion Strategies subheading.

16. Select one of the problem-solving methods listed in Section 4. Describe how you would use the technique in your class by applying it to a specific lesson plan.

Answer should make reference to the Teaching Students to Discuss section, Model Good Problem-Solving Techniques subheading.

17. Identify a group discussion or interaction in class that did not progress in ideal fashion. Discuss the group dynamics that occurred during the interaction. How did the dynamics affect the outcome of the discussion? How might they have been different? What could you have done to change the outcome?

Answer should make reference to the Teaching Students to Discuss section, Using Group Dynamics to Facilitate Discussion subheading and Group Techniques subheading.

18. Identify a situation in one of your classes that presented a barrier to discussion. Compare your handling of the situation to the techniques recommended in the module. Discuss what you would do the same in a similar situation as well as what you would do differently.

Answer should make reference to the Barriers to Discussion section.

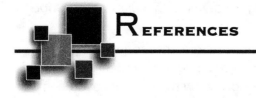

REFERENCES

Section 1: Effective Presentation Techniques

Adcox, J. (2001). *Does anybody remember playback anymore? Video fast forwards into the classroom.* Retrieved October 4, 2003, from University of California, Davis, IT Times Web site: http://ittimes.ucdavis.edu/spring2003/stories/Video3.htm

Buskist, W. & Saville, B. K. (2001). Creating positive emotional contexts for enhancing teaching and learning. *APS Observer, (March),* pp. 12–13, 19. Retrieved June 14, 2002, from http://www.socialpsychology.org/rapport.htm

From presenting to lecturing: Adapting material for classroom delivery. (2001). Retrieved June 14, 2002, from University of Waterloo, Teaching Resources and Continuing Education (TRACE) Web site: http://www.adm.uwaterloo.ca/infotrac/newtip.html

Section 2: Effective Listening Techniques

Davis, C. M. (1998). *Patient practitioner interaction: An experiential manual for developing the art of health care* (3rd ed.). Thorofare, NJ: SLACK, Inc.

Section 3: Effective Questioning Techniques

Bloom, B. (Ed.). (1956). *Taxonomy of educational objectives: The cognitive domain.* New York: Longmans, Green, & Co.

Cotton, K. (1988). Classroom questioning. *Northwest Regional Educational Laboratory School Improvement Research Series.* Retrieved July 7, 2003, from http://www.nwrel.org/scpd/sirs/3/cu5.html

Section 4: Effective Lecture Techniques

Royse, D. (2001). *Teaching tips for college and university instructors: A practical guide* (pp. 60–63, 103). Boston: Allyn and Bacon.

Vischeck simulates colorblind vision. (2002). Retrieved July 7, 2003, from http://www.vischeck.com

Section 5: Effective Discussion Techniques

Beaudin, B. (1999). Keeping online asynchronous discussions on topic. *Journal of Asynchronous Learning Networks, 3*(2).

Davis, B. G. (2001). *Tools for teaching* (pp. 63–81). San Francisco: Jossey-Bass.

McKeachie, W. J. (1999). *Teaching tips: Strategies, research, and theory for college and university teachers* (10th ed.) (Chapter 5). Boston: Houghton Mifflin Company.

Teaching by discussion. (1992). Retrieved July 7, 2003, from The Pennsylvania State University Center for Excellence in Learning & Teaching Web site: http://www.psu.edu/celt/newsletter/ID_Dec92.html

Yalom, I. D. (1975). *The theory and practice of group psychotherapy* (2nd ed.). New York: Basic Books, Inc.

Resources

Beaudin, B. (1999). Keeping online asynchronous discussions on topic. *Journal of Asynchronous Learning Networks, 3*(2).

Buskist, W. &. Saville, B. K. (2001). Rapport-building: Creating positive emotional contexts for enhancing teaching and learning. *APS Observer, 14*(3).

Champagne, D. (1995). *The intelligent professor's guide to teaching*. Pembroke, FL: ROC EdTech Publishing.

Christensen, C. R., Garvin, D. A., & Sweet, A. (Eds.). (1991). *Education for judgment: The artistry of discussion leadership*. Boston: Harvard Business School.

Cotton, K. (1988). Classroom questioning. *Northwest Regional Educational Laboratory School Improvement Research Series*. Retrieved July 7, 2003, from http://www.nwrel.org/scpd/sirs/3/cu5.html

Dantonio, M. & Beisenherz, P. C. (2000). *Learning to question, questioning to learn: Developing effective teacher questioning practices*. Needham Heights, MA: Allyn & Bacon.

Davis, B. G. (2001). *Tools for teaching*. San Francisco: Jossey-Bass.

Davis, J. R. (1976). *Teaching strategies for the college classroom*. Boulder, CO: Westview Press.

From presenting to lecturing: Adapting material for classroom delivery. (2001). Retrieved June 14, 2002, from University of Waterloo, Teaching Resources and Continuing Education (TRACE) Web site: http://www.adm.uwaterloo.ca/infotrac/newtip.html

Hyman, R. T. (1996). Questioning in the college classroom. Idea Paper No. 8. Manhattan, KS: Kansas State University Center for Faculty Evaluation and Development in Higher Education

Lowman, J. (1984). *Mastering the techniques of teaching*. San Francisco: Jossey-Bass.

McKeachie, W. J. (1999). *Teaching tips: Strategies, research, and theory for college and university teachers* (10th ed.). Boston: Houghton Mifflin Company.

Penner, J. G. (1984). *Why many college teachers cannot lecture*. Springfield, IL: Charles C. Thomas Publisher, Ltd.

Syllabus: Technology for higher education. (2003). Retrieved July 7, 2003, from http://www.syllabus.com

Teaching tips. (2003). Retrieved July 7, 2003, from The University of California, Santa Barbara, Office of Instructional Consultation Web site: http://www.id.ucsb.edu/IC/TA/tips/ta_tips.html

Teaching tips. (2003). Retrieved July 7, 2003, from University of Nebraska, Lincoln, Office of Graduate Studies Graduate Student Academic & Professional Development Web site: http://www.unl.edu/gradstud/GSAP/Teachingtips.html

Teaching tips index. (2003). Retrieved July 7, 2003, from Honolulu Community College Faculty Development Web site: http://www.hcc.hawaii.edu/intranet/committees/FacDevCom/guidebk/teachtip/teachtip.htm